Advancing DSM

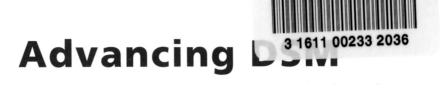
Dilemmas in Psychiatric Diagnosis

W9-BHM-735

Advancing DSM

Dilemmas in Psychiatric Diagnosis

Edited by

Katharine A. Phillips, M.D.
Michael B. First, M.D.
Harold Alan Pincus, M.D.

Published by the
American Psychiatric Association
Washington, D.C.

Note: The authors have worked to ensure that all information in this book is accurate at the time of publication and consistent with general psychiatric and medical standards, and that information concerning drug dosages, schedules, and routes of administration is accurate at the time of publication and consistent with standards set by the U.S. Food and Drug Administration and the general medical community. As medical research and practice continue to advance, however, therapeutic standards may change. Moreover, specific situations may require a specific therapeutic response not included in this book. For these reasons and because human and mechanical errors sometimes occur, we recommend that readers follow the advice of physicians directly involved in their care or the care of a member of their family.

The findings, opinions, and conclusions of this report do not necessarily represent the views of the officers, trustees, or all members of the American Psychiatric Association. The views expressed are those of the authors of the individual chapters.

Copyright © 2003 American Psychiatric Association
ALL RIGHTS RESERVED

Manufactured in the United States of America on acid-free paper
07 06 05 04 03   5 4 3 2 1
First Edition

Typeset in Adobe's Janson Text and Frutiger

American Psychiatric Association
1400 K Street, N.W., Washington, DC 20005
www.psych.org

Library of Congress Cataloging-in-Publication Data
Advancing DSM: dilemmas in psychiatric diagnosis / edited by Katharine A. Phillips, Michael B. First, Harold Alan Pincus.—1st ed.
      p. ; cm.
   Includes bibliographical references and index.
   ISBN 0-89042-293-1 (alk. paper)
   1. Mental illness—Classification. 2. Mental illness—Diagnosis. 3. Diagnostic and statistical manual of mental disorders. I. Phillips, Katharine A. II. First, Michael B., 1956- III. Pincus, Harold Alan, 1951-
   [DNLM: 1. Mental disorders—diagnosis. 2. Psychiatry—trends. WM 141 A2447 2002]
   RC455.2.C4 A384 2002
   616.89′075—dc21

                                                                2002027687

British Library Cataloguing in Publication Data
A CIP record is available from the British Library.

Contents

Contributors

Eric D. Caine, M.D.
John Romano Professor and Chair, Department of Psychiatry, University of Rochester Medical Center, Rochester, New York

Lynn Elinson, Ph.D.
Chief, Surveillance, Statistics and Research, NIOSH/Pittsburgh Research Laboratory, Department of Psychiatry, University of Pittsburgh School of Medicine, Pittsburgh, Pennsylvania

Robert N. Emde, M.D.
Professor of Psychiatry, University of Colorado Health Sciences Center

Stephen V. Faraone, Ph.D.
Associate Professor, Harvard Medical School Department of Psychiatry at Massachusetts General Hospital and Harvard Institute of Psychiatric Epidemiology and Genetics; Director of Research, Pediatric Psychopharmacology Service, Massachusetts General Hospital, Boston, Massachusetts

Michael B. First, M.D.
Research Psychiatrist, New York State Psychiatric Institute; Associate Professor of Clinical Psychiatry, Columbia University College of Physicians and Surgeons, New York, New York

Reed D. Goldstein, Ph.D.
Clinical Assistant Professor of Psychiatry, University of Pennsylvania School of Medicine, Philadelphia, Pennsylvania

Benjamin D. Greenberg, M.D., Ph.D.
Associate Professor of Psychiatry and Human Behavior, Brown University School of Medicine; Chief of Outpatient Services, Butler Hospital, Providence, Rhode Island

Alan M. Gruenberg, M.D.
Professor, Department of Psychiatry and Human Behavior, Jefferson Medical College; President, Gruenberg & Summers, P.C., Philadelphia, Pennsylvania

Steven E. Hyman, M.D.
Provost, Harvard University; Professor of Neurobiology, Harvard Medical School, Cambridge, Massachusetts

K. Ranga Rama Krishnan, M.B., Ch.B.
Professor and Chair, Department of Psychiatry and Behavioral Sciences, Duke University Medical Center, Durham, North Carolina

W. John Livesley, M.D.
Professor, Department of Psychiatry, University of British Columbia, Vancouver, British Columbia, Canada

Laurie E. McQueen, M.S.S.W.
Associate Director, Association Governance, American Psychiatric Association, Washington, D.C.

Katharine A. Phillips, M.D.
Associate Professor of Psychiatry and Human Behavior, Brown University School of Medicine; Director, Body Dysmorphic Disorder Program, Butler Hospital, Providence, Rhode Island

Harold Alan Pincus, M.D.
Professor and Executive Vice Chairman, Department of Psychiatry, Western Psychiatric Institute and Clinic, University of Pittsburgh School of Medicine; Senior Scientist, RAND; Director, RAND–University of Pittsburgh Health Research Institute, Pittsburgh, Pennsylvania

Lawrence H. Price, M.D.
Professor of Psychiatry and Human Behavior, Brown University School of Medicine; Clinical Director, Butler Hospital, Providence, Rhode Island

Steven A. Rasmussen, M.D.
Associate Professor of Psychiatry and Human Behavior, Brown University School of Medicine; Medical Director, Butler Hospital, Providence, Rhode Island

David Reiss, M.D.
Vivian Gill Distinguished Research Professor and Director, Center for Family Research, George Washington University Medical Center, Washington, DC

David C. Steffens, M.D., M.H.S.
Associate Professor, Department of Psychiatry and Behavioral Sciences, Duke University Medical Center, Durham, North Carolina

William S. Stone, Ph.D.
Assistant Professor of Psychology, Department of Psychiatry, Harvard Medical School, Massachusetts Mental Health Center; Training Coordinator, Harvard Institute of Psychiatric Epidemiology and Genetics, Boston, Massachusetts

Sarah I. Tarbox, B.A.
Research Assistant, Department of Psychiatry, Harvard Medical School, Massachusetts Mental Health Center, Boston, Massachusetts

Ming T. Tsuang, M.D., Ph.D., D.Sc., F.R.C.Psych.
Stanley Cobb Professor of Psychiatry and Psychobiology, Departments of Psychiatry & Epidemiology, Harvard University; Director, Harvard Institute of Psychiatric Epidemiology and Genetics, Boston, Massachusetts

Jerome C. Wakefield, D.S.W., Ph.D.
Professor, Institute for Health, Health Care Policy and Aging Research and the School of Social Work, Rutgers, the State University of New Jersey, New Brunswick, New Jersey

Foreword

Steven E. Hyman, M.D.

Psychiatric diagnosis is obviously crucial to clinical care, research, and public health, but it also has influences outside medicine—for example, in school systems and the criminal justice system. With the publication of the *Diagnostic and Statistical Manual of Mental Disorders*, 3rd Edition (DSM-III) (American Psychiatric Association 1980), psychiatric diagnosis in the United States took a major step forward. Building on the work of Robins and Guze (1970) and others, DSM-III reestablished the central significance of diagnosis in psychiatry, a significance that had been in question during the middle of the twentieth century, because psychoanalytic ideas had temporarily pushed the ideas of Kraepelin (1921/1976) off center stage. DSM-III powerfully reasserted the importance of diagnosis for treatment, prognosis, and research. It did much more, however, in the area of making diagnoses reliable. A major focus of DSM-III was the development and testing of criteria that would permit different clinicians or other trained observers to make the same diagnosis for the same patient. Although DSM-III and its successors—DSM-III-R (American Psychiatric Association 1987), DSM-IV (American Psychiatric Association 1994), and DSM-IV-TR (American Psychiatric Association 2000)—did not always succeed in providing criteria that would permit different diagnosticians to arrive at the same point (most notably in the area of personality disorders, as described by Livesley in Chapter 8 ["Diagnostic Dilemmas in Classifying Personality Disorder"]), attention to the issue of reliability is a great strength of the four manuals.

Overall, the approach of the four most recent DSMs is grounded in early evidence that mental disorders are disease entities that can be defined by operationalized sets of criteria based on symptoms and signs. It is difficult to overstate the importance for clinical care of replacing idiosyncratic diagnostic criteria with shared, operationalized criteria. With this change, a patient whose condition was diagnosed as schizophrenia in one hospital or clinic would very likely receive the same diagnosis in another, researchers would have increased assurance that they were investigating comparable patient groups, and treatment development could proceed with greater assurance.

Despite these successes, there are clear problems and unresolved controversies related to DSM-IV-TR, the most recent version of DSM. If a relative strength of DSM is its focus on reliability, a fundamental weakness lies in problems related to validity. Not only persisting but looming larger is the question of whether DSM-IV-TR truly carves nature at the joints— that is, whether the entities described in the manual are truly "natural kinds" and not arbitrary chimeras. The science of psychiatric disorders is still young, and thus psychiatric diagnosis must be expected to evolve as new scientific information emerges. The human brain is the most complex object in the history of scientific inquiry, and mental illness attacks aspects of brain function that represent the brain's highest levels of integration— cognition, emotion, and behavioral control (Hyman 2000). Moreover, risk of mental illness is based on an extraordinarily complex interplay of multiple genes, developmental events, and environmental influences, an interaction connoted by the term *genetic complexity* (Cowan et al. 2002). When DSM-III was published in 1980, the understanding of genetic complexity that dominates thinking about psychiatric disorders had not been formulated; neuroscience was just coalescing as a discipline; and important contemporary tools, such as functional magnetic resonance imaging, were yet to be invented.

I believe that psychiatry must ultimately have a diagnostic system based on pathogenesis, as is the case in the rest of medicine, but such a system remains in our future. I think that genetics, clinical neuroscience, behavioral science, and longitudinal clinical description will ultimately play critical roles in psychiatric diagnosis. Given emerging examples such as Alzheimer's disease, Parkinson's disease, hypertension, and diabetes, it appears likely that mental disorders (including depression, schizophrenia, panic disorder, and attention-deficit/hyperactivity disorder [ADHD]) will each represent clusters of illnesses with overlapping or even distinct genetic and nongenetic risk factors that converge to produce patterns of pathogenesis, symptoms, and course that have a close family resemblance.

The early nature of psychiatrists' understanding of psychiatric disorders is highlighted, perhaps unintentionally, in the excellent chapter by Steffens and Krishnan (Chapter 4, "Laboratory Testing and Neuroimaging"). This chapter is a well-wrought primer on diagnostic testing, but it is almost entirely abstract. Except for IQ tests to diagnose mental retardation and polysomnography to diagnose sleep disorders (polysomnography was inexplicably excluded from DSM-IV-TR criteria sets), diagnostic tests for mental disorders do not yet exist. When they are developed, such tests likely will have genetic, cognitive, and neuroimaging components. They are unlikely to involve peripheral measurements in serum or blood (except insofar as cells are a source of genetic material), because mental disorders represent abnormal functioning of neural circuits.

Without genotypes, objective tests, clues to pathogenesis, and even adequate family and longitudinal studies for most current diagnoses, it was not possible to establish a true empirical base for valid diagnoses in DSM-III, DSM-III-R, DSM-IV, and DSM-IV-TR. Instead, DSM-III was developed by a series of processes involving consensus. The degree of consensus was a remarkable achievement given the diverse and even combative theoretical orientations in psychiatry. That achievement notwithstanding, no one should mistake expert consensus for the truth. The possibility of gaining consensus—and broad adoption of the DSM system—derived in part from promulgation of the notion that the system was based on straightforward observations and had been cleansed of theoretical biases about etiology. However, any classification system must contain theory-based choices, even if they are not transparent. Moreover, a classification system based on a still young science lacks the full complement of empirical data that would reduce guesswork and obviate the need for some value-laden choices. Such nonempirical choices are reflected in the overall structure of DSM-III and its successors. Examples include the multiaxial approach to diagnosis (see Chapter 7, "Multiaxial Assessment in the Twenty-First Century"), the large-scale groupings of diagnoses (see Chapter 3, "Should the DSM Diagnostic Groupings Be Changed?"), the particular diagnoses chosen for inclusion, and, sometimes more interestingly, those chosen for exclusion. (In this regard, it is instructive to note that homosexuality was added as a diagnosis in DSM-III, in the absence of any significant empirical studies.)

The consensus agreements that resulted in these choices are not explained in the text. Some sections of DSM-III, DSM-III-R, DSM-IV, and DSM-IV-TR incorporate diverse theoretical positions, sometimes in awkward juxtaposition. As Livesley points out in Chapter 8 ("Diagnostic Dilemmas in Classifying Personality Disorder"), the placement of personality disorders on a separate diagnostic axis (Axis II) was meant to attract the attention of clinicians and researchers. It is not clear whether this was successful (very little high-quality research into personality disorders has been conducted [Hyman 2002]), but certainly it moved considerations other than science to the forefront. In addition, as Livesley argues, a major problem for clinicians is "the poor correspondence between DSM-IV-TR...diagnostic categories" for personality disorders and "typical presentations." In fact, Axis II in DSM-IV-TR contains a hodgepodge of putative diagnostic entities derived from sources ranging from family studies of schizophrenia (schizotypal personality disorder) to psychoanalytic theory (narcissistic personality disorder). Borderline personality disorder, an entity defined by empirical studies of symptom patterns, was so named because of an outdated theoretical position that it represents the border between neurotic and psychotic disorders.

The problems with Axis II bring to mind the larger question of whether a multiaxial system should be retained at all in DSM-V. A multiaxial approach has the laudable goal of achieving full, rich, and integrated clinical descriptions of individuals with psychiatric disorders, but other disciplines of medicine use the medical history for this purpose. As discussed by Gruenberg and Goldstein in Chapter 7 ("Multiaxial Assessment in the Twenty-First Century"), the multiaxial system has not, on the whole, been effectively used in psychiatric practice. Thus, designating certain portions of the assessment as axes may not only be unjustified scientifically but also lack clear real-world advantages for practice. Gruenberg and Goldstein propose elements of a multidimensional assessment that could be adopted in the future to combine diagnostic assessment with factors about the individual patient that might be important in treatment, prognosis, and management. However, in a manual focused on diagnosis, it is difficult to produce ancillary axes or dimensions that work well with the full panoply of diagnostic entities. For example, it is not clear why issues such as early trauma, as proposed by Gruenberg and Goldstein—which would of course be an important part of a medical history—should be recorded as a standard part of a diagnostic system, except in cases in which it was part of the pathogenesis, as in posttraumatic stress disorder (PTSD). Although given short shrift here, the question of whether to retain multiple axes, at least as they exist in DSM-IV-TR, will be a significant part of discussions leading to DSM-V.

One important, ongoing debate in personality disorders research that Livesley addresses concerns how a categorical approach to diagnosis (i.e., the idea that a disorder represents a syndrome with an identifiable separation from normalcy) can be made to work for behavioral traits that appear to be continuously distributed in the population (i.e., appear to be dimensional) and do not necessarily correlate with one another (i.e., are orthogonal dimensions). He argues that the categorical approach to personality disorders in DSM-IV-TR leads to arbitrary diagnostic decisions and, in turn, to the fact that most patients who qualify for any personality disorder diagnosis qualify for several personality disorder diagnoses. This question of a categorical versus dimensional approach to personality disorders remains both significant and unresolved.

Beyond personality disorders, one could raise questions about the current application of a simple categorical approach even for certain Axis I disorders. Numerous Axis I disorders may represent entities in which arbitrary cut points have been superimposed on continuous variables. This concern is exemplified by the threshold for a diagnosis of major depression (Kendler and Gardner 1998)—that is, by the fact that five of nine DSM-IV criteria must be present for at least 2 weeks. (This very issue was addressed by Andrew Solomon [2001] in *The Noonday Demon*, a book by a person with depression and intended for the general reader, thus serving to remind psychiatrists of the effect that perceptions of their diagnostic system has beyond their profession.) The use of cut points based on arbitrary measures of symptoms, chronicity, or severity to define the threshold of a disorder has important implications for treatment and reimbursement and has created a penumbra of controversial "subthreshold" psychiatric disorders. Pincus and colleagues, in Chapter 6 ("Subthreshold Psychiatric Disorders"), consider the status of these subthreshold disorders at length. Their concerns are closely related to consideration of the boundary between disorder and nondisorder described by Wakefield and First in Chapter 2 ("Clarifying the Distinction Between Disorder and Nondisorder"). An important goal in the development of DSM-IV was to set thresholds sufficiently high to avoid inclusion of ordinary problems of living as psychiatric disorders. However, setting thresholds too high might serve to deny preventive services or clinical care to individuals with early symptoms and substantial risk, including many children.

In medicine, this problem has increasingly been dealt with, where possible, through assignment of boundaries between normal states, high-risk states, and disorders on the basis of empirical studies of risk (National High Blood Pressure Education Program 1997; Vasan et al. 2002). Blood pressure in the population is a continuously distributed trait; the threshold for defining high blood pressure was assigned using results of long-term follow-up studies in which blood pressures above a certain cut point were associated with increased risk of stroke and myocardial infarction. These cut points have an empirical basis and were recently revised (see the introduction to National High Blood Pressure Education Program 1997; available at http://www.nhlbi.nih.gov/guidelines/hypertension/jncintro.htm). Specifically, the criteria for systolic hypertension worthy of treatment have been revised downward.

The case of cholesterol is in some ways even more illuminating (National Cholesterol Education Program 2002). Higher levels (but not extremely high levels) of low-density lipoprotein (LDL) cholesterol are considered not manifestations of an illness but a risk factor for cardiovascular disease. The level of desirable cholesterol has moved steadily downward, not only because of epidemiological studies of risk but also because of the development of relatively tolerable drugs (the statins) that decrease LDL cholesterol levels very effectively. Thus, boundaries of illness can be addressed by empirical studies of risk or harm, and thresholds for intervention can be addressed by empirical studies of disease-related risk versus the risks and benefits of the intervention. Psychiatric diagnosis would benefit from empirically established (rather than "consensus") thresholds both for disorders and for levels of risk that warrant current and evolving pharmacological or psychosocial interventions.

Clinical observations that at least some symptom complexes may represent continuous variables have dovetailed in recent years with progress in understanding genetic and other risk factors for psychiatric disorders—not only for mood and anxiety disorders but also for ADHD; autism; and, if Tsuang and colleagues (Chapter 5, "Insights From Neuroscience for the Concept of Schizotaxia and the Diagnosis of Schizophrenia") are right, schizophrenia. The actual relationship of genotypes to phenotypes must ultimately be established empirically; nonetheless, given the complex nature of risk of psychiatric disorders, it might be proposed that disorders represent continuous phenotypes based on the "dose" and "mixture" of risk-conferring genetic variants (risk alleles) and developmental and environmental risk factors. This complexity at the level of risk factors also heightens concerns about how to separate one disorder from another. Thus, for example, mood and anxiety disorders frequently co-occur (Kendler et al. 1987); there are individuals with schizophrenia, bipolar disorder, and schizoaffective disorder in the same pedigrees (Berrettini 2000); and obsessive-compulsive disorder (OCD), tic disorders, and ADHD frequently co-occur (see Chapter 3, "Should the DSM Diagnostic Groupings Be Changed?").

The high frequency of comorbidity may reflect different patterns of aggregation of multiple risk factors. Unfortunately, at this point one can only speculate about the underlying causes. Before speculation can be replaced by science, it is necessary first to identify a large number of genetic variants and environmental factors that produce risk of mental illness, and then to investigate how different numbers and mixtures of risk factors correlate with disease phenotypes. This already difficult task is further complicated by the fact that brain development depends on the *hierarchical* expression of many genes in interaction with the environment; thus it is unlikely that simple additive models of gene dosage will prove to be adequate explanations. Moreover, with regard to behavior, models created with the assumption that one gene causes one trait seem absurd today. One will therefore not be able to explain comorbidity by assuming that someone inherited a depression gene and an anxiety gene. Rather, both traits likely depend on multiple, and perhaps overlapping, risk factors.

DSM-IV-TR has numerous divisions in addition to axes. The manual contains 16 large groupings of diagnoses: 1) disorders usually first diagnosed in infancy, childhood, or adolescence, 2) delirium, dementia, and amnestic and other cognitive disorders, 3) mental disorders due to a general medical condition, 4) substance-related disorders, 5) schizophrenia and other psychotic disorders, 6) mood disorders, 7) anxiety disorders, 8) somatoform disorders, 9) factitious disorders, 10) dissociative disorders, 11) sexual and gender identity disorders, 12) eating disorders, 13) sleep disorders, 14) impulse control disorders not elsewhere classified, 15) adjustment disorders, and 16) personality disorders. Of these, personality disorders is also an axis (Axis II); the remaining 15 groupings are not directly related to any of the axes.

There has been little empirical justification for the groupings. In Chapter 3 ("Should the DSM Diagnostic Groupings Be Changed?"), Phillips and colleagues point out that the current, rather arbitrary groupings may produce unwanted consequences by falsely suggesting that certain disorders share risk factors or pathogenic processes. This impression of shared pathogenesis has clinical implications, in that the idea might falsely suggest shared approaches to treatment. A specific example in Chapter 3 raises questions about the large grouping of "anxiety disorders." OCD is currently classified as an anxiety disorder. However, there is increasing evidence that OCD, tic disorders such as Tourette's disorder, and body dysmorphic disorder are related. Several research groups (Graybiel and Rauch 2000; Leckman and Riddle 2000) have suggested that OCD and Tourette's disorder represent abnormalities in closely related or overlapping corticostriatal circuits. By this reasoning, OCD might be better grouped with Tourette's disorder—not with panic disorder and PTSD, which may reflect different abnormalities in amygdala-based fear circuitry (Gorman et al. 2000; Rauch et al. 2000). These alternative groupings of current anxiety disorders remain hypothetical but could be empirically researched with imaging studies of the neural circuits involved in these disorders.

Genetic studies also raise questions about the current large groupings of anxiety disorders. Some family studies suggest that generalized anxiety disorder and major depression may share risk genes (Kendler et al. 1987). If these disorders prove to be etiologically related, generalized anxiety disorder might be removed from its current grouping with panic disorder and PTSD and placed with mood disorders. The difficulty at this moment in history is that many of the problems are coming into clearer focus but the scientific data needed to develop a fully adequate diagnostic system are lacking.

Although genetics, neuroimaging, and other tools of clinical neuroscience have not yet helped psychiatrists draw boundaries around disease phenotypes, new approaches based on cognitive neuroscience and other emerging disciplines are already helping investigators to ask more penetrating questions about the boundaries promulgated by DSM-IV-TR. For example, as mentioned earlier, Tsuang and colleagues argue in Chapter 5 ("Insights From Neuroscience for the Concept of Schizotaxia and the Diagnosis of Schizophrenia") that DSM-IV-TR does not draw the boundaries of schizophrenia appropriately, and indeed psychotic symptoms (traditionally the hallmark of schizophrenia) should not be considered the central feature of this illness. The authors' arguments for a broader entity that they describe as schizotaxia, of which schizophrenia would be the most severe expression, are too preliminary to be fully convincing, but such ideas serve a fundamentally important role in that they provoke questioning of even the best-established diagnoses.

In Chapter 9 ("Relationship Disorders Are Psychiatric Disorders"), Reiss and Emde raise the interesting question of whether relationship disorders exist. Clearly there are examples of severe harm (e.g., spouse or child abuse) that, at least in some cases, appear to be limited to a specific relationship. (In fact, too little is known about the relationship between antisocial personality disorder, substance abuse, and what Reiss and Emde call relationship disorders.) Although the issue is critically important, I would suggest a conceptualization in which the disorder is more emphatically kept in the individual, and thus psychiatry is kept more fully congruent with the rest of medicine. In many psychiatric disorders, the disorder is separated from a conflict or a problem of living, in that symptoms are present across settings. Thus, for example, ADHD is not diagnosed if inattention, impulsivity, and hyperactivity are observed in the classroom but not at home or on the playground. In fact, however, the expression of certain disorders may be context dependent in the same way that angina pectoris may occur only if the person exceeds his or her exercise tolerance. With regard to psychiatric disorders, a pathogenic mechanism that may produce context dependence is associative learning, which has as its neural correlate synaptic remodeling. Associative learning may be the mechanism by which drug-related cues lead to resumption of drug use, even long after detoxification, in a person with addiction (Hyman and Malenka 2001); associative learning may also be the mechanism by which trauma-related cues elicit intrusive experiences in persons with PTSD. It is possible that what Reiss and Emde call relationship disorders are disorders in which associative-learning mechanisms (occurring against a background of risk factors) produce symptoms that are context dependent, in this case elicited by a specific person or persons.

To the extent that they encourage critical thinking and discussion, volumes such as this one are extremely important, given the enormous constraints on the evolution of a widely accepted diagnostic system. First, change is constrained because the DSM revision process remains one of consensus. Second, the manuals and their diagnostic criteria are widely disseminated, and the manuals have been adopted as guiding documents not only within psychiatry and the mental health professions but also within general medicine and law and even by the Food and Drug Administration, for use in consideration of appropriate indications for the development of new treatments.

Scientists interested in the classification of illness—and the framers of DSM-III, DSM-III-R, DSM-IV, and DSM-IV-TR—have known well that the strength of the current classification is reliability. Yet clinicians and even scientists attempting to discover genetic or neural underpinnings of disease have all too often reified the disorders listed in DSM-IV-TR as "natural kinds." This reification of DSM diagnostic entities has, in turn, created historical inertia in rethinking the nature and classification of psychiatric disorders. The science of mental illness is rapidly evolving, and critical to continued progress are studies relevant to pathogenesis and treatment that involve truly informative phenotypes. When investigators perform an imaging experiment, they recruit patients with DSM-IV-TR schizophrenia or major depression. In general, they do not question whether a valid phenotype is chosen when a DSM-IV-TR diagnosis is made, nor do they question how heterogeneous are the etiologies that produce a similar clinical picture. In reifying DSM-IV-TR diagnoses, one increases the risk that science will get stuck, and the very studies that are needed to better define phenotypes are held back.

The contributors to this volume present different perspectives, all aimed at addressing problems in diagnosis. Each author recognizes that despite its strengths, the current DSM-IV must be seen as a provisional diagnostic system. Because problems with DSM-IV are faced every day by clinicians (problems such as the high frequency of comorbidity or the intellectual incoherence of Axis II), debates about the DSM revision process should be made known to practitioners and should not be limited to arcane discussions within journals focused on nosology. The authors of this book demonstrate that fundamental thinking about psychiatric diagnosis is alive and well; and with the publication of the book, the nonspecialist can now read about many central concerns.

References

American Psychiatric Association: Diagnostic and Statistical Manual of Mental Disorders, 3rd Edition. Washington, DC, American Psychiatric Association, 1980

American Psychiatric Association: Diagnostic and Statistical Manual of Mental Disorders, 3rd Edition, Revised. Washington, DC, American Psychiatric Association, 1987

American Psychiatric Association: Diagnostic and Statistical Manual of Mental Disorders, 4th Edition. Washington, DC, American Psychiatric Association, 1994

American Psychiatric Association: Diagnostic and Statistical Manual of Mental Disorders, 4th Edition, Text Revision. Washington, DC, American Psychiatric Association, 2000

Berrettini WH: Are schizophrenic and bipolar disorders related? a review of family and molecular studies. Biol Psychiatry 48:531–538, 2000

Cowan WM, Kopnisky KL, Hyman SE: The human genome project and its impact on psychiatry. Annu Rev Neurosci 25:1–50, 2002

Gorman JM, Kent JM, Sullivan GM, et al: Neuroanatomical hypotheses of panic disorder, revised. Am J Psychiatry 157:493–505, 2000

Graybiel AM, Rauch SL: Toward a neurobiology of obsessive-compulsive disorder. Neuron 28:343–347, 2000

Hyman SE: Mental illness: genetically complex disorders of neural circuitry and neural communication. Neuron 28:321–323, 2000

Hyman SE: A new beginning for research on borderline personality disorder. Biol Psychiatry 51:933–935, 2002

Hyman SE, Malenka RC: Addiction and the brain: the neurobiology of compulsion and its persistence. Nat Rev Neurosci 2:695–703, 2001

Kendler KS, Gardner CO: Boundaries of major depression: an evaluation of DSM-IV criteria. Am J Psychiatry 155:172–177, 1998

Kendler KS, Heath AC, Martin NG, et al: Symptoms of anxiety and symptoms of depression: same genes, different environments? Arch Gen Psychiatry 44:451–457, 1987

Kraepelin E: Manic-Depressive Insanity and Paranoia. Translated by Barclay RM. Edited by Robertson GM. Edinburgh: Livingstone, 1921. Reprint, New York, Arno, 1976

Leckman JF, Riddle MA: Tourette's syndrome: when habit-forming systems form habits of their own? Neuron 28:349–354, 2000

National Cholesterol Education Program: Third Report of the Expert Panel on Detection, Evaluation, and Treatment of High Blood Cholesterol in Adults (Adult Treatment Panel III): Full Report. Available at: http://www.nhlbi.nih.gov/guidelines/cholesterol/atp3_rpt.htm. Accessed May 20, 2002

National High Blood Pressure Education Program: The Sixth Report of the Joint National Committee on Prevention, Detection, Evaluation, and Treatment of High Blood Pressure. Arch Intern Med 157:2413–2446, 1997 (Full report available at: http://www.nhlbi.nih.gov/guidelines/hypertension/jcintro.htm. Accessed August 1, 2002)

Rauch SL, Whalen PJ, Shin LM, et al: Exaggerated amygdala response to masked facial stimuli in posttraumatic stress disorder: a functional MRI study. Biol Psychiatry 47:769–776, 2000

Robins E, Guze SB: Establishment of diagnostic validity in psychiatric illness: its application to schizophrenia. Am J Psychiatry 126:983–987, 1970

Solomon A: The Noonday Demon: An Atlas of Depression. New York, Scribner, 2001, p 20

Vasan RS, Beiser A, Seshadri S, et al: Residual lifetime risk for developing hypertension in middle-aged women and men: the Framingham Heart Study. JAMA 287:1003–1010, 2002

Acknowledgments

The editors would like to thank John Rush, M.D., for his initial conception, implementation, and support of this project. The editors would also like to acknowledge the scientific and administrative contributions made to this volume by the following staff of the American Psychiatric Association: Yoshie Davison, Natalie Ivanovs, Tina Marshall, Ph.D., Laurie McQueen, M.S.S.W., and Sarah Tracy.

Introduction

Katharine A. Phillips, M.D., Michael B. First, M.D.,
Harold Alan Pincus, M.D.

In this book the authors present a number of diagnostic dilemmas that are mind-bending in their theoretical and scientific complexity and of utmost practical importance in everyday clinical decision making. Diagnosis and classification in psychiatry can easily be considered dry, arcane, and too sterile for a conflict-laden word such as *dilemma* to apply. However, as we strive to show in this volume, the term *dilemma* is very fitting because the diagnostic issues addressed here are unresolved and rife with controversy. These issues are important not only to researchers interested in classification but also to clinicians, because making an accurate diagnosis is the foundation for selecting the best treatment, determining prognosis, and enhancing understanding of the patients clinicians treat.

As Hyman notes in his Foreword to this volume, DSM was a landmark achievement for the field of psychiatry. By allowing diagnoses to be made in a reliable way, it has brought a great deal of order out of chaos and has fostered groundbreaking advances in both research and clinical care. For example, the operationalized diagnostic criteria introduced by DSM have made possible the recent explosion of research on empirically based psychological and pharmacological treatments. The criteria have also played a critically important role in the equally exciting progress now being made in clinical neuroscience. Without the ability to make reliable diagnoses—without DSM—such work would be severely hampered, if not impossible.

At the same time, many fundamental questions and controversies about the classification system remain. We have selected dilemmas for this book that were raised during the development of DSM-IV (American Psychiatric Association 1994), remain unresolved, and are certain to be revisited during the revision process leading to DSM-V. We hope that this book will stimulate further research into these controversial classification issues and, in turn, lead to improvements in future editions of DSM.

The authors of this book—leading researchers and clinicians in the field—tackle some of the larger, big-picture diagnostic dilemmas that the classification system faces. The focus of the initial chapters is on overarching topics that pertain to all of DSM, and specific examples are used to illustrate the selected dilemma. In Chapter 1 ("Determining Causation in Psychiatry"), Caine discusses the complex issue of how causality is determined in psychiatry, and he focuses on the issues involved in ascertaining whether a psychiatric syndrome is due to a general medical condition. He shows how approaches to determining causality in nonpsychiatric fields of medicine may be relevant to understanding causality in psychiatry, and he illustrates this idea with the hotly debated question of whether fen-phen causes psychopathology.

In Chapter 2 ("Clarifying the Distinction Between Disorder and Nondisorder"), Wakefield and First focus on an issue at the very heart of DSM: What is the definition of *mental disorder*, and how can this definition be used to help differentiate between mental (psychiatric) disorders and normal problems of living? The authors present a definition based on the concept of "harmful dysfunction"—that is, for something to be considered a disorder, it must both represent a dysfunction in some biological or psychological function of the brain and lead to significant harm to the individual. They then propose that this definition may be useful in reducing potential false positives (i.e., reducing the possibility of mislabeling problems of living as mental disorders).

In the next chapter (Chapter 3, "Should the DSM Diagnostic Groupings Be Changed?"), Phillips and colleagues argue that some of DSM's larger diagnostic groupings (e.g., the somatoform disorders) need to be reorganized and would be more valid if they were based on disorder etiology and pathophysiology (although the understanding of these things is admittedly limited). They propose, for example, that the category of "obsessive-compulsive–spectrum disorders," consisting of disorders currently scattered throughout DSM, may have more validity and clinical utility than some of the current diagnostic groupings.

Steffens and Krishnan, in Chapter 4 ("Laboratory Testing and Neuroimaging"), discuss the implications of laboratory testing and neuroimaging for psychiatric diagnosis and practice, using Alzheimer's disease as an example. Such tests are scarcely mentioned in DSM-IV-TR (American Psychiatric Association 2000), yet they are used routinely in other branches of medicine and hold remarkable promise as guides for diagnosing mental disorders.

In Chapter 5 ("Insights From Neuroscience for the Concept of Schizotaxia and the Diagnosis of Schizophrenia"), Tsuang and colleagues discuss how advances in neuroscience may change the diagnosis of schizophrenia. They reveal limitations of this disorder's criteria and propose an alternative conceptualization of schizophrenia, one based on the concept of schizotaxia.

Using minor depression as an example, Pincus and colleagues (Chapter 6, "Subthreshold Mental Disorders") illustrate the complexities of attempting to categorize subthreshold conditions. They highlight the need to consider the perspectives of primary care physicians and mental health specialists, as well as the risks of proliferation of different "brand names" for these conditions. They also suggest potential nosological and research strategies.

In Chapter 7 ("Multiaxial Assessment in the Twenty-First Century"), Gruenberg and Goldstein present a rethinking of the current five-axis system and a proposal for a new system that covers a wider range of domains. They argue that this alternative multiaxial system would better assist clinicians in developing a comprehensive understanding of their patients.

Livesley, author of Chapter 8 ("Diagnostic Dilemmas in Classifying Personality Disorder"), then tackles complex debates about the classification of personality disorders: Should personality disorders continue to be classified on a separate axis? Should DSM retain its current categorical approach or incorporate a dimensional structure? Should alternatives to current personality disorder diagnoses be used—alternatives that are more consistent with conceptions of normal personality and, Livesley argues, with the evidence?

In the last chapter (Chapter 9, "Relationship Disorders Are Psychiatric Disorders"), Reiss and Emde illuminate the important yet sorely neglected topic of relationship disorders and cogently argue that the disorders' clinical importance, as well as the available evidence, warrants their inclusion in DSM.

These are particularly challenging—and awkward—times for psychiatric nosology. For many reasons—scientific, clinical, policy—DSM has never been more important. Yet, as DSM becomes increasingly empirically based, one becomes more aware of the limitations of psychiatric knowledge. At the same time, empirical evidence that might advance DSM is dramatically increasing. A challenge we face is deciding when this evidence attains the critical mass required for making changes in DSM, especially in some of the broad, sweeping ways discussed in this book. This question is particularly relevant, and even more complex, if we ultimately revamp our classification system so that it is based on etiology and pathophysiology, as some authors recommend. The question for the next few editions of DSM is whether there will be enough data to make radical changes, since these manuals will take shape during a time when our knowledge of psychopathology will take a quantum leap forward. We hope that this book comes at just the right time to spur interest and research in preparation for the next iteration of DSM.

Katharine A. Phillips, M.D.

Michael B. First, M.D.

Harold A. Pincus, M.D.

References

American Psychiatric Association: Diagnostic and Statistical Manual of Mental Disorders, 4th Edition. Washington, DC, American Psychiatric Association, 1994

American Psychiatric Association: Diagnostic and Statistical Manual of Mental Disorders, 4th Edition, Text Revision. Washington, DC, American Psychiatric Association, 2000

CHAPTER 1

Determining Causation in Psychiatry

Eric D. Caine, M.D.

Contexts and Perspectives

Most psychiatric disorders are idiopathic conditions with no known causes. The literature is filled with debate about what constitutes a disorder or how one defines a case. Critics question the validity of current diagnostic classifications or nosologies, challenging their fundamental assumptions or theoretical underpinnings (Follette and Houts 1996). Because there is no method for externally validating current diagnostic constructs (i.e., verifying their accuracy using external measures that do not depend on the constructs themselves), it is likely that the field will be rife with controversy until the causes that lead to the emergence of specific clinical conditions can be determined.

In this chapter, I consider clinical reasoning processes that may provide a foundation for determining causation as it applies to psychiatric disorders. Rather than review specific theories of causation, however, I focus on the thought processes by which one weighs available evidence or draws conclusions regarding probable disease causation. At present, the task of determining causation relates most often to substance-induced disorders or psychiatric disorders due to a general medical condition, but such reasoning also should apply to proposed etiologically related conditions such as posttraumatic stress disorder (PTSD). Additionally, molecular neuroscience is beginning to clarify the complex interactions that underpin fundamental neurobiological processes and integrated brain functioning; as well, investigators will need to characterize the profound effects of brain-shaping environmental influences. Much of this work lies within the purview of genetic epidemiology (Kaprio 2000). In the years ahead, when more is known about the interactions of environmental and genetic risk factors associated with psychiatric disturbances, it will become necessary to determine the contributions of these factors to the expression of psychopathology. In the absence of definitive information regarding causation, one is nonetheless faced with a proliferation of presumed psychiatric diagnostic entities. Do these additions to each new edition of DSM reflect an enhanced understanding of real disease processes? How many of them are culturally bound manifestations of daily distress? What causes them? How can one understand these causal influences in a fashion that will facilitate effective therapeutics?

Before considering how one might determine causation among conditions that are now "idiopathic" disorders, it is important to reflect first on causal reasoning as it applies to substance-induced disorders or psychiatric disorders due to a general medical condition—that is, disorders in which an etiological tie between disease state and clinical presentation is explicit. In retrospect, one can observe that defining "rules" to determine causation for DSM-IV (American Psychiatric Association 1994) proved to be a difficult proposition indeed, one that may not have been entirely satisfying. It was not possible at that time to develop definitive criteria for including or excluding a condition. Appreciating the historical context of this continuing challenge will be critical in considering how to move into an era of correlating advances in genomics and proteomics with clinical phenomena and in seeking to understand causal associations. During the past quarter century, American "establishment psychiatry" has tried to steer away from its earlier practice of explaining the genesis of psychopathological conditions using psychoanalytic theory or its close relatives. Although specific theoretical notions were explicitly eschewed in DSM-IV, and DSM-III-R (American Psychiatric Association 1987) and DSM-III (American Psychiatric Association 1980) before it, clearly each edition was organized as a medical nosology, with the goals of promoting understanding of clinical presentation, natural history and prognosis, and treatment. This approach has been intensely criticized by some (Follette and Houts 1996). Although the recent DSM tradition has reaffirmed a disease orientation, it has not facilitated research to validate its constructs except through a series of "cross-validation" approaches and inferential methods, first laid out by E. Robins and Guze (1970) and later amplified by Kendell (1989). These remain inherently limited, indirect methods.

Invoking causes, conditions, and diagnoses identifies one immediately as ascribing to a medical model of disease and disorder. This model is based on defining deviations from optimal health or from normative functioning, which are complementary, not identical, concepts. Espousing a medical model does not mean that one considers biological processes or brain mechanisms the sole determinants of disease. Medical reasoning involves weighing and integrating psychological, social, and cultural determinants of causation, as well as elucidating potential biological routes of pathogenesis or symptom expression. A definable disease entity with a well-established cause need not be viewed only in biological terms. Environmental influences distinctly change brain function during the first months to years of life, or when, for example, a child learns cultural values, language, or the names of the 50 states. No doubt environmental influences or life circumstances can have etiological significance. In this chapter, *etiology* is defined as conditions or factors that cause or contribute to the development of a medical disorder. Pathogenic (or pathogenetic) mechanisms, for purposes of this discussion, are routes by which dysfunction or disease develops.

It is critically important to recognize the complex nature of determining causation. Fundamental to this dilemma is the challenge of establishing what disease is, clarifying the broader social and cultural construct "illness," and creating criteria or obtaining sufficient evidence to enable one to determine the causes of disease and illness. Psychiatric disorders, like other medical conditions, may involve either normal or abnormal physiological processes. How one labels these conditions, however, depends on one's understanding of the terms *disease* and *illness*.

For example, an individual may develop deviant behaviors to an extreme, perhaps disabling, degree, mediated by intact brain neurochemistry and brain physiology. That is, one can use the intact physiological processes of the brain to learn or develop a variety of traits, beliefs, or "abnormal" behaviors. Society and medicine may define these as illnesses, although there are no specifically associated pathobiological processes. (Indeed, it is especially important to appreciate the role of social and cultural values in the definition of these processes.) Conversely, the readily apparent disrupted brain functioning manifested by radical and sudden changes in sleep and circadian rhythms, appetite, thinking, and feeling that develops after a life event (such as the death of a parent, spouse, or child) is not classified as a psychiatric disorder. Even when all the "clinical" stigmata of profound disturbance are recognized, such a condition is not labeled as an illness until a lengthy interval has passed. Brain dysfunction that leads to disease may be inborn (e.g., Down syndrome or Huntington's disease [HD]) or acquired (e.g., severe trauma injury), permanent (e.g., the effects of a penetrating missile wound or a destructive lesion) or transient (e.g., alcohol intoxication), progressive (e.g., dementia due to Alzheimer's disease) or static (e.g., cognitive and behavioral deficits due to in utero exposure to alcohol). These categories need not be exclusive of one another. Additionally, however structurally static a lesion may be, its "illness effects" can be dynamic, because they have a ripple effect on the developmental course of an individual's life.

Typically, one considers how brain disorders lead to behavioral disturbances. This inside-to-outside view is central to current psychiatric thinking. However, it is just as important to recognize how interpersonal, environmental, or social events change the brain, either transiently (e.g., an acute stress response) or permanently (e.g., the formation of lasting memories). This outside-to-inside view must be investigated to understand how life experiences are a key to discerning individual differences at biological levels of expression (e.g., at the levels of proteomics or neurotransmitter functioning).

Diagnoses and Causal Reasoning

Diagnoses

Wulff (1976) described four types of diagnoses: symptom diagnoses, syndromes, anatomically defined conditions, and etiological diagnoses. *Symptom* or *pseudoanatomical diagnoses*, such as fever, headache, or chronic diarrhea, offer nothing to the clinician in terms of communicating information regarding treatment and prognosis. *Syndromes*—aggregated clusters of symptoms that probabilistically coexist—are empirically derived diagnoses whose utility is ultimately defined by their predictive validity, especially in terms of practical therapeutic utility. Given the absence of a test to ensure the accuracy of syndromic psychiatric conditions, clinicians must recognize that these conditions may reflect more than one etiology or pathogenic mechanism (Caine and Lyness 2000). DSM-IV is replete with syndromes that have not been validated. Although the use of explicit categorical criteria to define a case may enhance reliability, it is impossible to determine at this time whether such an approach in fact enhances or limits diagnostic validity. Indeed, one might seek to "test" all DSM-IV diagnoses by their predictive validity (i.e., their ability to predict responses to therapeutic interventions and prospectively frame the probabilities of longer-term clinical outcomes).

Anatomical diagnoses became the norm for much of general medicine during the nineteenth century, the great era of postmortem examination and clinical correlation. However, such methods have been shown to have limited utility in psychiatry. Moreover, organ- or tissue-related diagnoses (e.g., cirrhosis, cardiomyopathy, the characteristic pathology of Alzheimer's disease, and—until recently—all cancers) can have multiple etiologies, a situation that can be likened to the nonspecificity of syndromes. Such a perspective also underscores the emptiness of the "brain versus environment" debate that has entrapped generations of theorists and clinicians in psychiatry, psychology, and neurology. It is no surprise that all emotional and behavioral conditions involve brain functioning. Demonstrating that a condition is organic has little utility clinically unless there is a definable cause that can be treated; most often, clinicians are relegated to using treatments that were developed empirically for phenomenologically similar idiopathic psychiatric conditions. Ultimately, one must discern how brain function, psychological processes, and environmental influences interact to affect the expression of distress, disease, health, and illness.

Etiological diagnoses are based on causes, not manifestations. Thus, etiologically specific conditions cut across syndrome boundaries (called points of rarity by Kendell [1975]) and often organ system boundaries. For example, infectious and inflammatory-immune diseases and diabetes present with a wide array of symptoms, signs, or abnormal laboratory test results. Taken out of an integrative etiological context in centuries past, these clinically varied presentations were classified as separate disorders. Later, tests and studies determined their uniting causal mechanisms.

Clinicians in medicine use three complementary approaches to case reasoning: pathobiological, categorical, and individual (Caine and Lyness 2000). These methods are integrated by their utility in defining a patient's functional abilities and limitations. Establishing a diagnosis involves categorical case reasoning. Like any categorical process or classification method, clinical diagnosis (particularly the more approximate syndromic or anatomical diagnoses) relies on suppressing individual variation while highlighting common features. This key quality, the source of its generalized utility, also is the basis of many of its limitations.

Even when a physician understands the etiological route or routes of a condition, individual variations or differences profoundly influence the expression of disease and dysfunction. Too often, clinicians cloak their ignorance of the factors affecting individual differences in the expression of a disease by using vague terms such as *susceptibility, vulnerability,* or *resistance* or by elaborating theoretically appealing but generally unproven differences in immunity, state of mind, or social support. No doubt, understanding what protects and promotes health in the face of pathogenic exposures will be as important as understanding how disease develops, but at this time, the tendency is to focus on discovering group similarities rather than individual differences.

Causal Reasoning

There are three types of causal relationships, as depicted in Figure 1–1: necessary, sufficient, and contributory (Wulff 1976). In a *necessary condition,* a specific clinical state is always preceded by a unique etiology, but that etiology can lead to other disorders as well (e.g., tertiary syphilitic infection is necessary for general paresis with parenchymal brain involvement, but it also leads to meningovascular inflammation with its attendant findings, or to aortitis). A *sufficient cause* alone can engender a specific presentation, but other causes may lead to the same manifestations (e.g., HD and temporal lobe epilepsy both are sufficient to cause a schizophrenia-like psychotic syndrome). A *contributory cause* can lead to a specific presentation but does not do so uniformly, and there are other causes as well (e.g., traumatic brain injury can cause an amnestic disorder, but that outcome does not follow every instance of brain injury, and amnestic disorders also can be caused by herpes encephalitis).

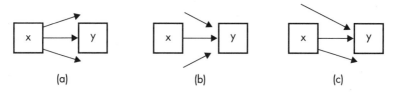

FIGURE 1–1. Different types of causal relationships.

(a) x is a necessary condition of y because y is always preceded by x. (b) x is a sufficient condition of y because x is always succeeded by y. (c) x is a contributory condition of y because x is sometimes succeeded by y, and y is sometimes preceded by x.

Source. Reprinted from Wulff HR (ed.): *Rational Diagnosis and Treatment.* Oxford, UK, Blackwell Scientific, 1976, p. 53. Used with permission.

Frequently, difficult-to-discern situations are encountered, and determination of causal relationships must be inferential. Psychiatry is not alone in this dilemma; these issues have been addressed in other fields of medicine for more than a century. The tradition of developing criteria for causal reasoning has been well described by others (Evans 1993), and its modern roots are in the rapidly developing nineteenth-century field of bacteriology. This tradition was inaugurated with the Henle-Koch postulates, which were added to, shaped, revised, and further revamped throughout the twentieth century, as new agents—such as viruses, prions, and most recently the human immunodeficiency virus—were discovered (Evans 1993).

Occupational and environmental medicine also have confronted similar quandaries, being faced with the challenge of understanding the relationships between workplace exposures (e.g., asbestos, motor vehicle exhaust, lead, pesticides) and the development of conditions that also occur in the general population, albeit less commonly. Practitioners of occupational medicine have struggled to assess causation even when an explicit mechanism of action tying etiology to clinical manifestations cannot be defined. These issues spill over into legal settings (with the law seeking to establish causal ties) and public health debates (about the possibility that expensive interventions may be necessary to reduce the occurrence of broadly based, preventable diseases).

For example, the crusade to reduce cigarette smoking grew from the causal reasoning methods used by the U.S. surgeon general in 1964 (Evans 1993; Hill 1965) and by others. Hill (1965), for instance, articulated two key questions: "How...do we detect these relationships between sickness, injury and conditions of work? How do we determine what are physical, chemical and psychological hazards of occupation, and in particular those that are rare and not easily detected?" (p. 295) Hill described nine aspects or qualities of association between two variables that may be helpful in determining a causal link. These aspects of association are strength, consistency, and specificity of association; temporality; biological gradient; plausibility; coherence; experiment; and analogy.

In this chapter, I review two scenarios that offer opportunities to "test" approaches to causal reasoning. The first involves a putative substance-induced cause of neuropsychiatric disturbances, the diet-drug combination fen-phen (fenfluramine and phentermine), which received professional, popular, and legal attention during the past decade. The fen-phen issue permits the use of Hill's (1965) guidelines, as well as those developed in recent legal forums for determining causation. The second scenario, involving the psychopathology associated with HD, allows assessment of the assumptions regarding the tie between genetic substrate and clinical manifestations, as well as a clear view of the limitations of the inferential reasoning approaches of Evans (1993) and Hill (1965).

Two "Test" Scenarios

Fen-Phen: Possible Cause of Psychopathology?

Is the reasoning process outlined by Hill (1965) helpful when one is trying to decide whether a putative exposure or environmental circumstance "causes" a psychiatric disorder? Stated in another fashion, when challenged with case reports or assertions about a psychiatric condition that is said to have a specific etiology, how does one "test" this issue using available clinical and experimental data? Rather than discuss a condition such as Alzheimer's disease (a substantial body of literature already exists regarding the psychopathology that can be ascribed directly to the actions of the disease [Jeste and Finkel 2000]), I consider if there is sufficient evidence to establish whether fenfluramine, dexfenfluramine, or their combination with phentermine caused clinically significant behavioral neurotoxicity, as manifested by diagnosed psychiatric disturbances among patients taking these medications as part of a weight reduction program. Similar to assertions regarding proposed causal relationships between the use of fluoxetine or isotretinoin and suicide, it was reported in the popular press, after publication of case reports in psychiatry journals, that the readily available diet-drug combination caused changes in mental state, depression, psychosis, and other neuropsychiatric disorders. This became a focus of litigation in federal and state courts.

In such instances, clinicians and scientists are often asked to offer opinions about disease causation, even when the scientific literature has not yet addressed the issue directly or identified a pathobiological mechanism of action. Although its immediate relevance to everyday psychiatry is limited (given manufacturer and Food and Drug Administration decisions to prohibit the use of the fen-phen combination), consideration of the psychopathogenic capability of this combination involves the same type of testing or reasoning processes that will be applicable in the future for deciding whether there are specific genes that contribute to the expression of particular psychiatric conditions—indeed, whether there is sufficient proof to establish a causal relationship.

As stated earlier, Hill (1965) described nine aspects or qualities of association: strength, consistency, and specificity of association; temporality; biological gradient; plausibility; coherence; experiment; and analogy. (Often it seems that strength and consistency are difficult to dissociate; they might therefore be subsumed under the term *robustness*.) Although these qualities may serve as useful benchmarks, they may be more usefully arrayed in some type of format that makes sense within the spectrum of knowledge about pathophysiological processes and clinical symptoms and signs. Regarding fen-phen, one can establish four categories for such an analysis: neurotoxicology, the neurobiology of psychiatric disorders, epidemiology, and clinical psychopathology. This approach is akin to that taken during recent litigation concerning silicone breast implants, when court-appointed experts reviewed the basic toxicology of silicone, the pertinent clinical immunology and relevant epidemiology, and related clinical rheumatology (Diamond et al. 1998).

Neurotoxicology

There is substantial suggestive evidence that fenfluramine, dexfenfluramine, and their combination with phentermine cause neurotoxic brain damage in a variety of test animal species (Appel et al. 1989; Halladay et al. 1998; Harvey et al. 1977; Kalia 1992; Kleven and Seiden 1989; Lee et al. 1997; McCann et al. 1994; Miller and O'Callaghan 1994; Molliver and Molliver 1990; O'Callaghan and Miller 1994; Ricaurte et al. 1991; Rowland 1994; Rowland et al. 1993; Sanders-Bush et al. 1975; Schechter 1990; Schuster et al. 1986; Westphalen and Dodd 1993a, 1993b; Wilson and Molliver 1994). However, there also is significant controversy in the literature; findings (and opinions) depend on the types of animals used, the dosages and routes of administration, the duration of exposure, and the experimental laboratory methods used to detect changes in neuronal elements. There is debate as well about whether drug-induced changes are permanent or transient (due to pharmacological actions) and whether damaged neurons can sprout portions after apparent "dying back" because of toxic effects. Indeed, there is debate about how to define neurotoxicity in these animal models and whether findings can be generalized to humans.

Despite elements of controversy in the literature, there is a strong trend toward reproducible occurrence of neurotoxic effects due to fenfluramine and dexfenfluramine, specifically effects targeting serotonin neurons. Although this conclusion is not sufficient to determine causality, it provides a plausible basis for exploring whether these medications caused clinically significant neuropsychiatric symptoms or signs in patients taking them for weight control.

Neurobiology of Psychiatric Disorders

The exact pathobiological (neurobiological) mechanisms for expression of psychopathological conditions remain unknown. However, substantial progress has been made during the past 20 years, and there are now a variety of good candidates to explain the brain mechanisms that mediate expression of distinct symptoms, signs, and syndromes. It is clear that deficiency of serotonin-mediated neurotransmission is associated with important clinical conditions, such as major depression, anxiety disorders, aggression, impulsive suicide attempts, and problems with spontaneity or initiation, sleep, and appetite (Charney et al. 1999). It remains to be determined what causes disruptions in serotonin neurochemistry, but there is little doubt that medications that enhance serotonin brain systems often lead to positive clinical improvements in affected psychiatric patients. This knowledge combined with the available information about the neurotoxic effects of fenfluramine and dexfenfluramine makes a proposed cause-and-effect relationship more plausible. Both current knowledge and theory also touch on coherence—that is, tying a proposed plausible mechanism to what is known about a particular disease.

Epidemiology

Hill (1965) presented *strength*, *consistency*, and *specificity of association* as the first three (and most important) elements linking an environmental exposure and a clinical condition in a cause-and-effect relationship. Each of these elements depends on an epidemiologically sound approach to defining the prevalence and features of a specific condition and how they relate to a potential etiology. However, no epidemiological studies have tied fen-phen exposure to any psychiatric disturbances. Without epidemiological findings, it is impossible to create a causal link between a proposed etiology and an array of clinical manifestations. One must establish these elements of the causal chain to integrate what is known about potential toxic or pathogenic mechanisms, as they are manifested in populations, with what one encounters in individual patients. Thus, clinical epidemiology is the context in which all other elements of reasoning must make sense; in other words, epidemiology serves as the bridge between proposed etiologies or disease mechanisms and potential manifestations.

Clinical Psychopathology

The available clinical literature is remarkably sparse. Nearly all reports are letters to the editor rather than reports of rigorous studies involving defined patient populations (Harding 1971, 1972; Hooper 1971; Myers et al. 1994; Preval and Pakyurek 1997; Raison and Klein 1997; Schenck and Mahowald 1996; Steel and Briggs 1972; Toornvliet et al. 1994). Even the report of the largest case series might be best described as an "organized anecdotal" report (McCann et al. 1998); the study failed to use standardized clinical diagnostic methods or uniform approaches to case history and reporting. No controlled studies matched affected individuals with others having similar key characteristics in order to determine possible distinctive features or risk factors. In contrast to investigations of reported cardiac defects after fen-phen use (Jick et al. 1998), no studies followed an at-risk (i.e., drug-exposed) population to determine who developed psychiatric symptoms or signs, and no studies compared the characteristics of affected individuals with those of unaffected individuals. The lack of such studies precludes the definition of a cause-and-effect relationship. A key element in any proposed toxic-exposure litigation is the diagnosis of proposed (i.e., contested) cases in light of what has been published or defined in the scientific literature. The fen-phen clinical literature is so sparse and the cases are so poorly documented that an expert would not be able to establish a similarity between contested cases and those described previously.

Comment

One cannot establish a cause-and-effect relationship between fen-phen exposure and the subsequent development of neuropsychiatric symptoms or signs. No doubt intriguing leads exist in the available data (McCann et al.

1997), but such hints and inklings fail to meet any standard of medical or scientific certainty or definable probability. Although the fen-phen issue draws on many of the aspects of association outlined by Hill (1965), four (temporality, biological gradient, experiment, and analogy) are not addressed specifically in this example but may play a role in other efforts to determine causation.

In a toxic-exposure situation, whether an adverse outcome of treatment with medications or an environmental or occupational exposure, one is often confronted with questions of how much and how long. Clinicians tend to look for dose-response effects when speaking of pharmacological actions. However, two apparently nontoxic compounds may interact with each other, and this interaction may lead to a toxic effect that precludes easy elaboration of a dose-response gradient or curve (Schaumburg and Spencer 1987). In other types of brain disorders, a linear relationship may not be a universal finding. A small isolated lesion that damages a key area may have devastating effects, and using the term *dose* does not always capture the quality of this type of injury. In addition, some observable clinical effects reflect crossing a threshold beyond which compensatory mechanisms are ineffective (e.g., the emergence of Parkinson's disease after loss of a requisite proportion of neurons in the substantia nigra). Beyond this threshold, response gradients may be less evident; indeed, one may encounter a dose-response ceiling (i.e., one may find that further exposure does not lead to a greater clinical effect).

Temporality also can be tricky. In its favor (and quite compelling in some instances), temporal association is intuitively sensible; that is, exposure is shortly followed by the emergence of signs and symptoms in a previously healthy individual. There is inherent face validity to this situation, although one certainly must guard against coincidental or chance occurrences. Thus, temporality is buttressed by strength, consistency, and specificity; alone it is greatly weakened. However, idiosyncratic adverse drug responses (for instance, agranulocytosis due to clozapine therapy) may be so rare and delayed that initial appraisals of temporal association or causal tie are inaccurate. Other examples also warn against drawing easy conclusions. Whereas the majority of toxins have their greatest effect at the time of highest exposure, radiation has a delayed effect; a neuropsychiatric condition due to cerebral irradiation may begin more than a year after treatment and may unfold gradually during the ensuing decade (Grossman et al. 1994). Similarly, psychosis due to temporal lobe epilepsy has been found to begin 5–10 years after the onset of the seizure disorder (Slater et al. 1963). And as noted in the next section ("Huntington's Disease: One Gene, Many Manifestations"), the psychopathological manifestations of HD may precede any evidence of movement disorder and cognitive impairment.

Experiment, though desirable, may be neither feasible nor ethical. Removal of a suspected but unproven toxic compound from an environment may be attempted experimentally in an ethical fashion; however, exposing individuals to an uncertain but suspected toxin cannot easily be justified. The twentieth century saw too many ethically unacceptable medical experiments that focused on disease causation and clinical manifestation, such as the Tuskegee Syphilis Study, the unknowing exposure of individuals to plutonium, and the Nazi cold water–immersion tests.

Analogy may clarify understanding but by itself indicates little regarding causation.

Huntington's Disease: One Gene, Many Manifestations

HD has been a subject of intensive psychopathological research. It begins largely in middle age and has the unique quality of being a single-gene disorder that can be diagnosed with a high degree of confidence on the basis of family history and a characteristic movement disorder (Harper 1996). Morphological and physiological changes in pathology are similarly revealed by computed tomography, magnetic resonance imaging (MRI), or positron emission tomography as by postmortem pathological examinations of the brain.

Even before the identification of the HD gene on chromosome 4 (Huntington's Disease Collaborative Research Group 1993) and the characterization of its abnormally expanded CAG repeats and the formation of abnormal huntingtin protein, investigators examined affected individuals and at-risk family members to characterize the phenomenology and epidemiology of psychiatric disturbances of patients and their relatives (Baxter et al. 1992; Caine and Shoulson 1983; Dewhurst 1970; Dewhurst et al. 1969; Di Maio et al. 1993; Folstein 1991; Folstein et al. 1983a, 1983b; Jensen et al. 1993, 1998; Lovestone et al. 1996; McHugh and Folstein 1975; Oliver and Dewhurst 1969; Shiwach 1994; Watt and Seller 1993). Taken together, these studies demonstrated that mood disturbances (both major and minor depression), psychotic states (including a schizophrenia-like syndrome), personality changes, and other psychiatric conditions occurred more frequently in HD gene carriers than in unaffected family members or in large community epidemiological samples (L. N. Robins and Regier 1991). Roughly speaking, 40% of HD patients have a mood disturbance and 10% have a psychotic disturbance. Perhaps 25% have no psychiatric symptoms beyond the characteristic dementia. Still to be determined is what distinguishes HD patients who develop clinically significant psychopathology from those who do not. The neuropsychological and motor abnormalities of HD occur in all of those affected, at least to some measurable degree, and these abnormalities have a common form in all patients with HD, although severity may vary (Bamford and Caine 1986).

HD presents a quandary to the DSM-using psychopathologist today, a dilemma described nearly two decades ago (Caine and Shoulson 1983). Our field now is in its second quarter century of a movement to define the biological and etiological underpinnings of psychiatric disorders by creating relatively homogeneous clinical clusters. This derives from the belief that strict syndrome boundaries are related to definably separate pathogenic mechanisms and, in turn, to distinct etiological processes. HD challenges this assumption. No factors have been identified that modify the expression of psychopathology in individuals carrying the HD gene. Some authors suggest that psychiatric presentations run true in families (Folstein et al. 1983a; Jensen et al. 1993), but this is not a universal finding. Although others argue that the number of CAG repeats may have an effect on the severity of the characteristic cognitive impairment (Jason et al. 1997), there is no indication of a similar effect on psychopathology.

The lessons of HD are clear. One could use a "test," following the guidance of authors such as Evans (1993) and Hill (1965), and demonstrate convincingly that HD causes an array of psychopathological disturbances—that it is a specific, apparently sufficient etiology among affected individuals. If there were an HD-like disorder that did not have the movement abnormalities and dementia to set it apart, or, more recently, a defined genetic abnormality, one would likely separate related patients into diverse and distinct clusters on the basis of clinical phenomena alone. Use of discriminating clinical criteria would lead one down a blind alley.

DSM-V and the Future

Although I have focused primarily on conditions with pathobiological bases, the same method of causal reasoning is equally applicable to psychologically or socially mediated etiological factors. Certainly this is a testable issue.

For example, one could examine available data to discern whether environmental factors, such as natural disasters, cause psychiatric disorders. As a first step, one would want to use epidemiological findings to determine what proportion of an exposed population developed a clinically significant disturbance. Certainly it would be necessary to define a threshold for establishing "caseness," taking into account criteria used in past community-based epidemiological surveys. At a minimum, the latter studies also should serve as the comparison standard for establishing whether affected communities or populations have increased rates of psychopathology. A prospectively collected comparison sample is optimal but may be unavailable or prohibitively expensive to collect.

Beyond measuring the frequency of conditions, one must define the array of presenting symptoms, signs, and syndromes. Most would probably fall into a depressed-anxious spectrum, with only a modest proportion conforming to stereotypically defined PTSD; there would be few (if any) individuals developing new-onset psychoses. If sufficient data are available, one should compare the findings from several disasters to assess the consistency as well as the specificity of these presentations. It also might be possible to determine a dose-response relationship, with the least-exposed individuals having fewer symptoms (or a lower proportion of symptoms fulfilling criteria for "cases") and the most-exposed persons (measured in a standard fashion) being the most greatly affected psychopathologically. One might find a dose-response ceiling; that is, there may come a point when more or greater exposure does not create any more pathology, perhaps because the vast majority of the population has been affected. But even under the most horrendous circumstances, some individuals do not show frank pathology. (It would be most helpful to understand what protects persons at risk who are not affected.) Beyond these parameters, it would be important to assess plausibility and coherence and to monitor the temporal relationship between being caught in a disaster and the subsequent emergence of symptoms and signs.

Once this analysis is completed, it should be possible to make reliable and valid statements regarding causation, or, at the very least, one could consider what missing data would be crucial for establishing either the presence or the absence of such a link. In contrast to the case-based clinical approach, this method involves combining population-based perspectives and testing a theory regarding a specific etiology; it does not depend on first refining a homogeneous patient cluster and then seeking the cause or causes of the patients' condition.

Turning again to biological mechanisms, let us take as an example efforts to tie suicide, attempted suicide, and impulsive behaviors to genes related to 5-hydroxytryptophan (serotonin) (a key to serotonin synthesis [Roy et al. 1997]) or to a serotonin receptor subtype (Du et al. 2000). Suppose that there were reproducible findings demonstrating a higher frequency of a hypothetical low–serotonin-synthesizing allele among men ages 25–50 years who have made medically dangerous suicide attempts or have completed suicide. Most of these individuals have comorbid depression and substance or alcohol use disorders (Conwell et al. 1996); many commit so-called impulsive suicides within a few hours to days or, at most, a few weeks after disruptive life experiences (Duberstein et al. 1993).

How are such genetics findings applied? Should this low–serotonin-synthesizing allele be labeled a suicide gene? Before publication of such a statement, which would be followed by media clamor, one would first want to establish the full array of clinical features and personal attributes associated with this allele, in both a variety of patient populations and unaffected community samples. No doubt one would want to avoid the traps associated with collection of samples from postmortem tissues alone or from subjects with psychiatric disorders or subjects who made serious suicide attempts. Although suicide among younger men is associated with impulsive traits, suicide among elderly persons is often planned with care and then carried out in an especially lethal fashion (Conwell et al. 1998). *Impulsive* is not an apt description for most older people who commit suicide. Additionally, impulsiveness is a characteristic of many people who exhibit neither suicidality nor psychopathology. Indeed, in the case of affectively stable individuals, one might consider attributes such as decisiveness rather than impulsiveness. It is unclear how to generalize from men to women, especially when considering suicide, since there appear to be important qualitative differences between men and women who complete suicide across all ages. Additionally, how should genetic findings be integrated with compelling epidemiological data that show substantial regional, national, and culturally related variations in suicide rates among both men and women? Do these variations reflect broad population fluctuations in the prevalence of the "suicide gene"? Perhaps, but one should be very cautious before concluding that there is a single gene that causes what seems to be such a multidetermined complex behavior.

Conclusion

In this chapter, I outlined approaches to case reasoning and causal determination that are not often used in psychiatry. These methods remain imperfect, although they may prove more satisfactory than those available to the writers of DSM-IV. Presently available data, however, often prove insufficient to support even these approaches. Additionally, modern American psychiatry has tended to downplay (however inadvertently) what is not known by creating an extraordinarily complex classification system, one that errs on the side of giving many variations of clinical presentation new diagnostic tags, even though it remains to be determined whether these variations presage differences in either treatment or prognosis. In contrast to recent nosological trends, Judd and Akiskal (2000) argued persuasively that there now is ample evidence to consider unipolar depression a spectrum of manifestations, viewed best across a dynamic clinical continuum of symptoms and signs that fluctuate or evolve throughout the patient's illness.

Thus, I advocate that a truly conservative approach be taken in the planning of DSM-V—not an approach that maintains the status quo, but one that tests current diagnostic entities for the rigor of the data that support them. Psychiatric disorders due to a general medical condition would at least need to undergo the type of scrutiny outlined by Hill (1965) or by Evans (1993), with the limitations of these methods being taken into account.

For example, an Australian colleague recently suggested that so-called vascular depression (Alexopoulos et al. 1997) be added to DSM-V as an etiologically specific subtype of depressive disorders (E. Chiu, personal communication, April 1999). This suggestion raised a number of questions. How much more common are vascular lesions—as detected by MRI, for example—in a population of elderly patients with later-onset depression than in a community-based control population? (Of course, the control group should have a truly normative distribution; it should not consist entirely of ideally healthy, highly educated subjects—individuals who tend to volunteer for medical research studies.) Is there a relationship between quantifiable cerebrovascular risk factors, MRI findings, and the occurrence of depression? (One might study populations high in the former, looking for definable associations between the latter two.) Are there a specific clinical presentation and course that separate the depressed patients with vascular lesions (depression in these patients typically begins later in life) from patients whose depression began at a similar age but who have no vascular lesions? Is there a temporal relationship between lesions and clinical manifestation? Is there a biological gradient relating dose to severity? (One should expect to detect evidence of either a cumulative effect of cerebral lesions or specific placement of lesions in key areas known to have a pathogenic effect.)

Until one had answered these questions, it would not be possible to thoughtfully address challenges such as plausibility and coherence. But today, the tendency is to deal with these latter issues first, often by discerning possible analogies, or putative associations based on subject groups drawn from extreme samples or created with selection biases, and then extrapolating from these nonrepresentative groups to propose potential etiologies of disease. Unfortunately, an emphasis on trying to discern etiological or mechanistic associations in small numbers of subjects leads to false conclusions that there are cause-and-effect ties. As a counterweight, the recommendations put forth by Hill (1965) or Evans (1993) can serve as bulwarks against the current emphasis on evidence-based medicine. Even as one engages in more rigorous "testing," however, it is crucial to remember that these are guidelines, not rules. Rothman and Greenland (1999) noted the limitations of Hill's approach. Surely the lessons of HD, a single-gene disorder with a variety of presentations, directly challenge notions such as consistency and specificity.

Despite these limitations, use of such yardsticks would likely mean a more parsimonious application of "due to" diagnoses in daily clinical practice. This type of approach can be used in either clinical practice or research settings (Conwell et al. 1996; Lyness et al. 1993). Rather than guessing at causation when there are insufficient data, one can note both Axis I and Axis III conditions and then define the disease burden and the functional limitations of the patients or research subjects that arise separately from the individuals' psychiatric disturbances and general medical conditions. This has proven to be a feasible method empirically, one that has effectively and reproducibly disentangled the effect of patients' comorbid conditions. For example, it is possible to assess the distinctive longer-term contributions of psychopathological and medical burdens to the ensuing clinical status of depressed inpatients (Lyness et al. 1993).

Thus, for DSM-V, all presumed etiologically related conditions (e.g., substance-induced psychotic disorder, PTSD, or adjustment disorders) should be tested in a fashion akin to the example of testing whether fen-phen causes psychopathology. Some disorders will stand up to such a test; others will be eliminated, likely for the better. For example, such a testing process may well demonstrate that most trauma-exposed individuals do not develop PTSD per se. But if these persons have a mood disturbance due to trauma, that too is revealing and apt to be therapeutically useful. Perhaps then one might reconsider current nosology, which is based on etiology rather than phenomenology. Although PTSD as a rubric speaks superficially to etiology, its current criteria force one to focus attention on a relatively specific pattern of symptoms and signs. Etiology is not uniquely associated with clinical phenomena. Thus, it remains to be defined whether the "PTSD" diagnosis of recent decades has shown demonstrable therapeutic or prognostic utility, or has resulted only in misleading pseudoprecision.

Of course, most conditions do not have causes that can be defined at this time. In medical parlance, they are idiopathic (e.g., idiopathic schizophrenia, idiopathic major depression, or even idiopathic antisocial personality). These are considered "primary" psychiatric disorders in DSM-IV-TR (American Psychiatric Association 2000). When causation cannot be determined, one must at least challenge each diagnostic construct using the inferential methods outlined by E. Robins and Guze (1970) and Kendell (1975, 1989). Does each diagnostic construct aid therapies and delineate distinctive prognoses? Put another way, what is the predictive validity of each construct?

As psychopathologists consider the causes of psychiatric disorders, they also must describe factors that protect individuals who encounter the same etiologically powerful insults (i.e., bear common risks) but do not develop any detectable disturbances. What spares these people? Such factors must be studied if one is to achieve the fullest understanding of the etiologies and pathogenic mechanisms that cause psychiatric disturbances—an understanding akin to the emerging appreciation regarding the multidetermined nature of cardiovascular diseases, cancers, and many infectious diseases. This task will require the same discipline of mind that is described in this chapter. Such discipline will be needed in the attempt to establish evidence-based causes of health (Evans 1978), a critical step when moving from what has often been palliative psychiatric care for patients with serious psychiatric disorders to new models of cure and prevention.

References

Alexopoulos GS, Meyers BS, Young RC, et al: 'Vascular depression' hypothesis. Arch Gen Psychiatry 54:915–922, 1997

American Psychiatric Association: Diagnostic and Statistical Manual of Mental Disorders, 3rd Edition. Washington, DC, American Psychiatric Association, 1980

American Psychiatric Association: Diagnostic and Statistical Manual of Mental Disorders, 3rd Edition, Text Revision. Washington, DC, American Psychiatric Association, 1987

American Psychiatric Association: Diagnostic and Statistical Manual of Mental Disorders, 4th Edition. Washington, DC, American Psychiatric Association, 1994

American Psychiatric Association: Diagnostic and Statistical Manual of Mental Disorders, 4th Edition, Revised. Washington, DC, American Psychiatric Association, 2000

Appel NM, Contrera JF, DeSouza EB: Fenfluramine selectively and differentially decreases the density of serotonergic nerve terminals in rat brain: evidence from immunocytochemical studies. J Pharmacol Exp Ther 249:928–943, 1989

Bamford KA, Caine ED: The neuropsychology of Huntington's disease: problems of clinical-pathological correlation in a progressive brain illness, in Advances in Clinical Neuropsychology, Vol 3. Edited by Tarter R, Goldstein G. New York, Plenum, 1986, pp 181–212

Baxter LR, Mazziotta JC, Pahl JJ, et al: Psychiatric, genetic, and positron emission tomographic evaluation of persons at risk for Huntington's disease. Arch Gen Psychiatry 49:148–154, 1992

Caine ED, Lyness JM: Delirium, dementia, and amnestic and other cognitive disorders, in Comprehensive Textbook of Psychiatry/VII, 7th Edition, Vol 1. Edited by Sadock BJ, Sadock VA. Baltimore, MD, Williams & Wilkins, 2000, pp 854–923

Caine ED, Shoulson I: Psychiatric syndromes in Huntington's disease. Am J Psychiatry 140:728–733, 1983

Charney DS, Nesler EJ, Bunney BS (eds): Neurobiology of Mental Illness. New York, Oxford University Press, 1999

Conwell Y, Duberstein PR, Cox C, et al: Relationships of age and Axis I diagnoses in victims of completed suicide: a psychological autopsy study. Am J Psychiatry 153:1001–1008, 1996

Conwell Y, Duberstein PR, Cox C, et al: Age differences in behaviors leading to completed suicide. Am J Geriatr Psychiatry 6:122–126, 1998

Dewhurst K: Personality disorder in Huntington's disease. Psychiatr Clin (Basel) 3:221–229, 1970

Dewhurst K, Oliver J, Trick KLK, et al: Neuro-psychiatric aspects of Huntington's disease. Confin Neurol 31:258–268, 1969

Diamond BA, Hulka BS, Kerkvliet NI, et al: Silicone breast implants in relation to connective tissue diseases and immunologic dysfunction: a report by a national science panel to the Honorable Sam C. Pointer Jr., coordinating judge for the Federal Breast Implant Multi-district Litigation. Available at: http://www.fjc.gov/BREIMLIT/SCIENCE/report.htm (15 December 1998). Accessed 12 August 2002

Di Maio L, Squitieri F, Napolitano G, et al: Suicide risk in Huntington's disease. J Med Genet 30:293–295, 1993

Du L, Bakish D, Lapierre YD, et al: Association of polymorphism of serotonin 2A receptor gene with suicidal ideation in major depressive disorder. Am J Med Genet 96:56–60, 2000

Duberstein PR, Conwell Y, Caine ED: Interpersonal stressors, substance abuse, and suicide. J Nerv Ment Dis 181:80–85, 1993

Evans AS: Causation and disease: a chronological journey. The Thomas Parran Lecture. Am J Epidemiol 108:249–258, 1978

Evans AS: Causation and Disease: A Chronological Journey. New York, Plenum, 1993

Follette WC, Houts AC: Models of scientific progress and the role of theory in taxonomy development: a case study of the DSM. J Consult Clin Psychol 64:1120–1132, 1996

Folstein SE: The psychopathology of Huntington's disease, in Genes, Brains, and Behavior. Edited by McHugh PR, McKusick VA. New York, Raven, 1991, 181–191

Folstein SE, Abbott MH, Chase GA, et al: The association of affective disorder with Huntington's disease in a case series and in families. Psychol Med 13:537–542, 1983a

Folstein SE, Franz ML, Jensen BA, et al: Conduct disorder and affective disorder among the offspring of patients with Huntington's disease. Psychol Med 13:45–52, 1983b

Grossman H, Caine ED, Ketonen L: Progressive irradiation dementia and psychosis. Neuropsychiatry Neuropsychol Behav Neurol 7:125–129, 1994

Halladay AK, Fisher H, Wagner GC: Interaction of phentermine plus fenfluramine: neurochemical and neurotoxic effects. Neurotoxicology 19:177–184,
1998

Harding T: Fenfluramine dependence. Br Med J 3:305, 1971

Harding T: Depression following fenfluramine withdrawal. Br J Psychiatry
121:338–339, 1972

Harper PS (ed): Huntington's Disease, 2nd Edition, Vol 31. London, WB Saunders, 1996

Harvey JA, McMaster SE, Fuller RW: Comparison between the neurotoxic and se-
rotonin-depleting effects of various halogenated derivatives of amphetamine in
the rat. J Pharmacol Exp Ther 202:581–589, 1977

Hill AB: The environment and disease: association or causation? Proc R Soc Med
58:295–300, 1965

Hooper AC: Fenfluramine and dreaming. Br Med J 3:305, 1971

Huntington's Disease Collaborative Research Group: A novel gene containing a
trinucleotide repeat that is expanded and unstable on Huntington's disease
chromosomes. Cell 72:971–983, 1993

Jason GW, Suchowersky O, Pajurkova EM, et al: Cognitive manifestations of Huntington's disease in relation to genetic structure and clinical onset. Arch Neurol
54:1081–1088, 1997

Jensen P, Sørensen SA, Fenger K, et al: A study of psychiatric morbidity in patients
with Huntington's disease, their relatives, and controls: admissions to psychiatric hospitals in Denmark from 1969 to 1991. Br J Psychiatry 163:790–797,
1993

Jensen P, Fenger K, Bolwig TG, et al: Crime in Huntington's disease: a study of reg-
istered offences among patients, relatives, and controls. J Neurol Neurosurg
Psychiatry 65:467–471, 1998

Jeste DV, Finkel SI: Psychosis of Alzheimer's disease and related dementias: diagnostic criteria for a distinct syndrome. Am J Geriatr Psychiatry 8:29–34, 2000

Jick H, Vasilakis C, Weinrauch LA, et al: A population-based study of appetite-sup-
pressant drugs and the risk of cardiac-valve regurgitation. N Engl J Med
339:719–724, 1998

Judd LL, Akiskal HS: Delineating the longitudinal course of depressive illness: beyond clinical subtypes and duration thresholds. Pharmacopsychiatry 33:3–7,
2000

Kalia M: Dex-fenfluramine when administered orally in doses in considerable excess of the human therapeutic dose produces no ultrastructural or axonal transport changes in raphe serotonergic neurons of the rat (abstract). Abstracts—
Society for Neuroscience 18, 1992

Kaprio JK: Genetic epidemiology. BMJ 320:1257–1259, 2000

Kendell RE (ed): The Role of Diagnosis in Psychiatry. Oxford, Blackwell Scientific,
1975

Kendell RE: Clinical validity. Psychol Med 19:45–55, 1989

Kleven MS, Seiden LS: D-, L- and DL-Fenfluramine cause long-lasting depletions
of serotonin in rat brain. Brain Res 505:351–353, 1989

Lee R, Weisenberg B, Vosmer G, et al: Combined phentermine/fenfluramine administration enhances depletion of serotonin from central terminal fields. Synapse 26:36–45, 1997

Lovestone S, Hodgson S, Sham P, et al: Familial psychiatric presentation of Huntington's disease. J Med Genet 33:128–131, 1996

Lyness JM, Caine ED, Conwell Y, et al: Depressive symptoms, medical illness, and functional status in depressed psychiatric inpatients. Am J Psychiatry 150:910–915, 1993

McCann U[D], Hatzidimitriou G, Ridenour A, et al: Dexfenfluramine and serotonin neurotoxicity: further preclinical evidence that clinical caution is indicated. J Pharmacol Exp Ther 269:792–798, 1994

McCann UD, Seiden LS, Rubin LJ, et al: Brain serotonin neurotoxicity and primary pulmonary hypertension from fenfluramine and dexfenfluramine: a systematic review of the evidence. JAMA 278:666–672, 1997

McCann UD, Eligulashvili V, Ricaurte GA: Adverse neuropsychiatric events associated with dexfenfluramine and fenfluramine. Prog Neuropsychopharmacol Biol Psychiatry 22:1087–1102, 1998

McHugh PR, Folstein MF: Psychiatric syndromes in Huntington's chorea: a clinical and phenomenologic study, in Psychiatric Aspects of Neurological Diseases. Edited by Benson DF, Blumer D. New York, Grune & Stratton, 1975, 267–286

Miller DB, O'Callaghan JP: Environment-, drug- and stress-induced alterations in body temperature affect the neurotoxicity of substituted amphetamines in the C57BL/6J mouse. J Pharmacol Exp Ther 270:752–760, 1994

Molliver DC, Molliver ME: Anatomic evidence for a neurotoxic effect of (±)-fenfluramine upon serotonergic projections in the rat. Brain Res 511:165–168, 1990

Myers JE, Mieczkowski T, Perel J, et al: Abnormal behavioral responses to fenfluramine in patients with affective and personality disorders: correlation with increased serotonergic responsivity. Biol Psychiatry 35:112–120, 1994

O'Callaghan JP, Miller DB: Neurotoxicity profiles of substituted amphetamines in the C57BL/6J mouse. J Pharmacol Exp Ther 270:741–751, 1994

Oliver JE, Dewhurst KE: Six generations of ill-used children in a Huntington's pedigree. Postgrad Med J 45:757–760, 1969

Preval H, Pakyurek AM: Psychotic episode associated with dexfenfluramine. Am J Psychiatry 154:1624–1625, 1997

Raison CL, Klein HM: Psychotic mania associated with fenfluramine and phentermine use (letter). Am J Psychiatry 154:711, 1997

Ricaurte GA, Molliver ME, Martello MB, et al: Dexfenfluramine neurotoxicity in brains of non-human primates. Lancet 338:1487–1488, 1991

Robins E, Guze SB: Establishment of diagnostic validity in psychiatric illness: its application to schizophrenia. Am J Psychiatry 126:983–987, 1970

Robins LN, Regier DA (eds): Psychiatric Disorders in America: The Epidemiologic Catchment Area Study. New York, Free Press, 1991

Rothman KJ, Greenland S: Causation and causal inference, in Modern Epidemiology, 2nd Edition. Edited by Rothman KJ, Greenland S. Philadelphia, PA, Lippincott-Raven, 1999, pp 7–28

Rowland NE: Long-term administration of dexfenfluramine to genetically obese (ob/ob) and lean mice: body weight and brain serotonin changes. Pharmacol Biochem Behav 49:287–294, 1994

Rowland NE, Kalehua AN, Li B-H, et al: Loss of serotonin uptake sites and immunoreactivity in rat cortex after dexfenfluramine occur without parallel glial cell reactions. Brain Res 624:35–43, 1993

Roy A, Rylander G, Sarchiapone M: Genetics of suicides: family studies and molecular genetics. Ann N Y Acad Sci 836:135–137, 1997

Sanders-Bush E, Bushing JA, Sulser F: Long-term effects of p-chloroamphetamine and related drugs on central serotonergic mechanisms. J Pharmacol Exp Ther 192:33–41, 1975

Schaumburg HH, Spencer PS: Recognizing neurotoxic disease. Neurology 37:276–278, 1987

Schechter MD: Functional consequences of fenfluramine neurotoxicity. Pharmacol Biochem Behav 37:623–626, 1990

Schenck CH, Mahowald MW: Potential hazard of serotonin syndrome associated with dexfenfluramine hydrochloride (Redux) (letter). JAMA 276:1220–1221, 1996

Schuster CR, Lewis M, Seiden LS: Fenfluramine: neurotoxicity. Psychopharmacol Bull 22:148–151, 1986

Shiwach R: Psychopathology in Huntington's disease patients. Acta Psychiatr Scand 90:241–246, 1994

Slater E, Beard AW, Glithero E: The schizophrenia-like psychoses of epilepsy. Br J Psychiatry 109:95–150, 1963

Steel JM, Briggs M: Withdrawal depression in obese patients after fenfluramine treatment. Br Med J 3:26–27, 1972

Toornvliet AC, Pijl H, Meinders AE: Major depression during dexfenfluramine treatment (letter). Int J Obes Relat Metab Disord 18:650, 1994

Watt DC, Seller A: A clinico-genetic study of psychiatric disorder in Huntington's chorea. Psychol Med (suppl 23):1–46, 1993

Westphalen RI, Dodd PR: New evidence for a loss of serotonergic nerve terminals in rats treated with d,l-fenfluramine. Pharmacol Toxicol 72:249–255, 1993a

Westphalen RI, Dodd PR: The regeneration of d,l-fenfluramine-destroyed serotonergic nerve terminals. Eur J Pharmacol 238:399–402, 1993b

Wilson MA, Molliver ME: Microglial response to degeneration of serotonergic axon terminals. Glia 11:18–34, 1994

Wulff HR (ed): Rational Diagnosis and Treatment. Oxford, Blackwell Scientific, 1976

CHAPTER 2

Clarifying the Distinction Between Disorder and Nondisorder

Confronting the Overdiagnosis (False-Positives) Problem in DSM-V

Jerome C. Wakefield, D.S.W., Ph.D., Michael B. First, M.D.

In this chapter, we focus on an issue that is at the heart of DSM: the definition of *mental disorder* and the distinction between disorders and other problems of living. Even an improved definition of *mental disorder*, however, will not solve all of psychiatry's nosological problems and will inevitably have many limitations. For example, it has been argued that any attempt to come up with a definition of *mental disorder* that adequately covers every conceivable scenario is doomed to fail (Frances et al. 1992). Moreover, no full, precise delineation of disorder (in contrast to nondisorder) should be expected, because almost every concept encompasses some fuzzy boundary cases in addition to clear cases on both sides of the boundary (Lilienfeld and Marino 1995; Wakefield 1996). Indeed, the text accompanying the DSM-IV-TR (American Psychiatric Association 2000) definition of *disorder* includes the following: "no definition adequately specifies precise boundaries for the concept of 'mental disorder'" (p. xxx). One could also argue that the inclusion of a comprehensive definition of *disorder*, though potentially desirable, is not required for a classification system to exist. For example, in the *International Statistical Classification of Diseases and Related Health Problems*, 10th Revision (ICD-10; World Health Organization 1992), the official classification system that covers all medical conditions, no attempt is made to define *disease* or *illness*. Furthermore, the definition of *mental disorder* in DSM-IV (American Psychiatric Association 1994) and DSM-IV-TR was adapted from a definition first introduced in

DSM-III (American Psychiatric Association 1980); DSM-I (American Psychiatric Association 1952) and DSM-II (American Psychiatric Association 1968) were constructed in the absence of such a definition. However, it has been argued that during inclusion and exclusion decisions, any such nosology relies on a distinction between disorders and other problems, so in fact there is always a concept of disorder involved, and the challenge is to make it more explicit and adequate (Wakefield 1992b).

Despite the potential limitations, the inclusion of a definition of *mental disorder* clearly offers some important advantages. First and foremost, the definition can help in the creation of a conceptual framework for delineating the boundaries between mental disorders and healthy states. Thus, such a definition provides guidance on how to construct diagnostic criteria sets for individual disorders so as to minimize overdiagnosis or the "false-positives" problem—that is, to prevent labeling as mental disorders conditions that represent nondisorder problems of living. This conceptual framework can also be of assistance in making decisions, during the DSM revision process, concerning whether newly proposed syndromes represent psychiatric disorders or nondisorder problems of living (e.g., whether road rage is a psychiatric disorder or an undesirable behavior). Even when it does not help in the assessment of new categories or the formulation of new criteria, a definition of *mental disorder* can help explain why particular distinctions are made and why there are disputes about some conditions. Finally, the definition can also be of help in distinguishing between mental disorders and other medical conditions. This latter advantage depends on clarifying what makes a disorder a mental disorder, whereas the advantages concerning false positives depend on clarifying what makes a psychiatric condition a disorder.

We first briefly consider how a definition of *mental disorder* may be useful in setting the boundary between mental disorders and other medical conditions. We do not address this problem in depth; we only comment on the nature of the problem and possible directions for a solution. We then turn to the more important question—and the main focus of this chapter—of how a definition of *mental disorder* can help solve the DSM-IV-TR false-positives problem by providing guidance for distinguishing disorders and nondisorders. We attempt to provide a systematic analysis of the problem and to formulate an improved approach.

Setting the Boundary Between Mental Disorders and Neurological Conditions

During the past several years, questions have been raised regarding whether certain disorders that are considered mental disorders in DSM-

IV-TR should be considered neurological conditions. For example, a request was submitted to the National Center for Health Statistics (which oversees the official United States implementation of the classification of diseases presented in ICD) to move Tourette's disorder, in the *International Classification of Diseases*, 9th Revision, Clinical Modification (ICD-9-CM; World Health Organization 1978), from the chapter titled "Mental Disorders" (Vol. 1) to the chapter titled "Diseases of the Nervous System and Sense Organs" (Vol. 1). Although the primary motivation for this move was to increase reimbursement for treatment of this condition (essentially sidestepping the parity issue), the evidence supporting the claim included functional imaging studies that demonstrated central nervous system dysfunction.

This imaging finding raises general, troubling questions for psychiatry. If many psychiatric disorders are based in central nervous system dysfunction, are they mental disorders or neurological disorders? Does this spell the end of psychiatry as a separate discipline, as psychiatric conditions become understood in terms of brain dysfunction and are reclassified as neural conditions? Can a serviceable distinction somehow be retained between psychiatric and neurological disorders?

There is no easy answer to these questions in current nosological practices. The general organizational principle governing the placement of disorders in larger categories in ICD-10 is rather ad hoc, being based on both etiology (e.g., the first two chapters are titled "Infectious and Parasitic Diseases" and "Neoplasms") and physiology or anatomy (e.g., "Endocrine, Nutritional, and Metabolic Diseases and Immunity Disorders," "Diseases of the Blood and Blood-Forming Organs," and "Diseases of the Genitourinary System"). These sorts of distinctions do not help much in drawing the boundary between neurological and mental disorders because both entail dysfunctions involving the central nervous system. Historically, the distinction between a mental disorder and a neurological condition has paralleled mind-body dualism: disturbances with an established physiological etiology localized to the central nervous system have been considered neurological, whereas idiopathic or functional disturbances have been deemed psychiatric. Thus, ignorance of brain pathology allowed many conditions to be considered psychiatric disorders, which later, as knowledge increased, became known as neurological disorders. For example, before the discovery of a physiological basis for seizures, epilepsy was considered a psychiatric condition. Now that it has been determined that the etiologies of many mental disorders have biological components, a boundary based on an organic/nonorganic division is no longer sensible.

However, some mental disorders might not involve neurological dysfunctions. Some dysfunctions may not be dysfunctions in neurological "hardware" but may instead be dysfunctions in the processing of psychological meanings that form the "software" of the brain. Consider an animal analogue: a gosling that accidentally imprints on a passing fox will die because it is fixated on following and staying close to the fox, and one might well consider this behavior a mental disorder in the gosling. Yet nothing has gone wrong with anything at the neurological-hardware level; the imprinting system has performed its function of psychologically attaching the gosling to the first creature it sees on hatching. The failure of natural function has to do with the fact that the imprinting mechanism has the function of attaching the gosling to its mother, and the imprinting mechanism has failed in this function because of an unanticipated accident. The imprinting mechanism depends on an expected and usually reliable environmental correlation between "mother" and "first creature seen on hatching." Search as one might, one will find no neurological disorder—that is, there is no disorder describable in terms of a dysfunction of neurological tissue without reference to representations and other psychological meanings. The neurological systems in the gosling's case are functioning as designed in terms of neurological-level descriptions. The problem lies in the fact that the stored representation is not a representation of the right object. We conclude that it is at least possible for some mental disorders to occur in the mental software of representational meanings without being reflected in any dysfunctions describable at the neurological-hardware level. However, this is likely not the case with many major mental disorders, which do appear to correspond to neurological dysfunctions.

It is often assumed that mental disorders are those with mental etiologies. That is not entirely correct. Consider, for example, psychosomatic illnesses, which were classified as mental disorders in DSM-II and largely reclassified as physical disorders (with psychological factors contributing to etiology) in DSM-III. The fact that a mental process caused a physical disorder did not mean that the resulting disorder was a mental disorder, because the resulting type of dysfunction was physical. If the psychological factor was itself an independently specifiable mental disorder, one would say that there are both a mental disorder and a physical disorder, and perhaps that the physical disorder is secondary to the mental disorder.

Such examples point to the fact that probably the most meaningful distinction between mental and nonmental involves the domain of disorder functions, not the etiology per se. A mental disorder involves a dysfunction in a cognitive, motivational, behavioral, emotional, or other psychological mechanism. Roughly, psychological mechanisms are those that have some special involvement of representational meanings or consciousness. Of course, some of the functions included in this list (e.g., cognition, intentional behavior) straddle the boundary between what is traditionally considered neurological and what is traditionally considered psychiatric. In many cases, whether a particular type of dysfunction is considered psychiatric or neurological reflects historical traditions regarding which specialty is primarily involved in its management. For example, aphasia secondary to a stroke (in the absence of other cognitive deficits) is traditionally considered neurological because patients with this condition are typically cared for by neurologists, whereas the syndrome of memory loss, loss of abstract reasoning, and personality change (symptoms that add up to dementia) is considered psychiatric because a psychiatrist is primarily responsible for management. Depending on the form and the person's ability to influence expression, abnormalities in movement (which are elements of behavior) may be considered neurological (e.g., choreiform movements) or psychiatric (tics). There seems to be an irreducible arbitrary element in such classification decisions that is not addressed by conceptual analysis alone. In principle, however, in terms of the logic of the concept *mental disorder*, any disorder in which a psychological function is impaired is a mental disorder, perhaps secondary to a physical disorder.

In the end, what is important is that dysfunctions are recognized and diagnosed, both at the neurological level and at the psychological level, and that such distinctions are not obscured by domain disputes between branches of medicine. The definition of *mental disorder* should highlight that what makes a disorder mental is the functional domain, not etiology. Most importantly, such concerns must not form an obstacle to integrating both psychological and biological factors in a unified understanding of etiology and multiple levels of dysfunction.

Ultimately, establishing the boundary between mental disorders and other general medical conditions is inherently much less important than clarifying the boundary between disorder and nondisorder. Whereas the classification of a condition as mental or neurological need have no implications for correct identification of the problem, confusion about the distinction between disorder and nondisorder can lead to false positives and/ or false negatives in diagnosis and to nonoptimal treatment decisions. Therefore, we focus in the rest of this chapter on the delineation between disorder and nondisorder.

Setting the Boundary Between Mental Disorders and Problems of Living

What are the boundaries between mental disorders and "normal" states or nondisorders? What role, if any, should distress or impairment play in distinguishing disorders from nondisorders? To what extent should social values be considered when defining disorders? These questions bear directly on the issue of how to formulate criteria sets that are specific to disorders and thus how to minimize false-positive diagnoses (i.e., classification of nondisorder conditions as disorders), an area of public and professional concern. After describing the nature, history, and importance of the false-positives problem, we consider the strengths and weaknesses of the DSM-IV-TR definition of *mental disorder* in terms of distinguishing disorders from normal states. We then propose, as a clarification and revision of the DSM-IV-TR definition, Wakefield's (1992a) analysis of *mental disorder* as a "harmful mental dysfunction," with harm being determined by social values and the word *dysfunction* referring to a failure of a mental mechanism to perform its natural (i.e., evolutionarily selected) function. This analysis appears to be consistent with the broader use of *disorder* in medicine. Finally, we survey ways of addressing the false-positives problem—ways involving refinement of criteria sets so that they are consistent with the harmful-dysfunction analysis—and suggest which strategies are the most promising and how they might be implemented in the revision process leading to DSM-V.

False-Positives Problem in DSM

From the perspective of DSM-V, one of the main motives for clarifying the concept of mental disorder is to help improve the ability to draw a distinction between mental disorder and nondisorder problems of living. The distinction needs clarification because the label "mental disorder" is often incorrectly applied to many other kinds of undesirable negative conditions that are not disorders. These conditions include normal intense emotional reactions, social deviance, conflict between an individual and social institutions, personal unhappiness, lack of fit between an individual and a specific social role or relationship or environment, and socially disapproved or negatively evaluated behavior in general. Thus, views that essentially equate disorders with socially disvalued nondisorder conditions (see, e.g., Ausubel 1971; King 1981; Kirmayer and Young 1999; Moore 1978; Pichot 1986; Sedgwick 1973, 1982) do not express the medical concept of disorder. Statistical unexpectedness (see, for example, Kendell 1975; Scadding 1967, 1990; Taylor 1971, 1976) and treatability (e.g., Kendell 1986; Lilienfeld and Marino 1999) have also often been considered indicative of a disorder but are not essential to the definition of *disorder* (Wakefield 1999b).

   The issue of whether the conceptual boundary of disorder has been overextended to include nondisorder problems of living is not new, but it has evolved into a new form. In the 1960s and 1970s, psychiatry was criticized vehemently by both professionals and nonprofessionals, who argued that there is no such thing as a "mental disorder" in the literal medical sense. Psychiatric diagnosis was claimed to be just a matter of medically labeling socially disvalued nondisorder conditions for purposes of social control. It was argued that psychiatrists could not reliably distinguish disorder from nondisorder or one purported disorder from another, which thus proved the invalidity of diagnostic concepts. These radical critiques, by noted thinkers such as Szasz (1974), Scheff (1966, 1975), Laing (1967), Sarbin (1967), and Foucault (1965, 1978), came to be known as the antipsychiatry movement.

There are many reasons why the antipsychiatry movement is no longer a potent force. One reason is that with the publication of DSM-III in 1980, many of the antipsychiatrists' criticisms were squarely and systematically addressed by the psychiatric community. DSM-III provided a definition of *mental disorder* that attempted to distinguish mental disorders in the medical sense from social deviance and other kinds of personal and social problems. Moreover, common nondisorder conditions that may warrant psychiatric attention were distinguished from disorders and listed separately in a section called "V Codes for Conditions Not Attributable to a Mental Disorder That Are a Focus of Attention or Treatment." Most importantly, DSM-III offered operationalized theory-neutral definitions of each disorder that improved reliability and contributed to valid differentiation of disorders from nondisorders and one disorder from another. These innovations, along with other developments such as the growth of evidence of a biological basis and effective pharmacological treatment for some disorders, have pretty much put the psychiatry critiques to rest. The claim that the concept of mental disorder is incomprehensible or that mental disorders do not exist is rarely heard these days except in postmodernist or radical behaviorist treatises and is not a major concern in public discourse about psychiatry.

Psychiatry now faces a new challenge regarding its basic concept of mental disorder, and we will argue that a comparably systematic assault on this challenge should be undertaken in the process of constructing DSM-V. The new challenge again comes both from within the mental health professions and from the lay public. The focus of this challenge is not on whether mental disorders exist at all but rather on whether mental health professionals, when using DSM criteria, are overdiagnosing in such a way that many other kinds of human problems are deemed pathological. This new challenge contains an echo of the old antipsychiatry concerns about social control and mislabeling of nondisorder conditions as disorders. However, it is much more subtle and targeted, and it is not inherently antagonistic to the broader goals and conceptual approach of psychiatry. The new challenge consists of a diverse set of objections to the labeling of specific conditions as disorders on a category-by-category basis. With a few exceptions, the complaint is that a particular category is being overextended, because of overinclusive diagnostic criteria, to encompass some nondisorder conditions as well.

We will call the criticism that the DSM criteria are overly inclusive the *false-positives problem.* By *false positives* we do not mean the haphazard application of DSM criteria, such as when an individual's condition is classified as a disorder even though the individual does not have a disturbance that meets DSM criteria for any disorder. Rather, false positives are understood here as nondisorder conditions that nevertheless are contained within the DSM criteria for a disorder. Ironically, the problem of false-positive diagnoses has become much more obvious and in certain ways more serious since the widespread acceptance of DSM's explicit operationalized criteria. So this new challenge is in a sense born of the success in meeting the previous antipsychiatry challenges. There is no implication that nondisorder conditions are necessarily less problematic or less worthy of attention or help; they are simply not mental disorders. And although a conceptual analysis of criteria can reveal potential false positives, the actual extent of false positives remains unknown.

Criteria that identify all individuals with disorders, and only individuals with disorders, are referred to as conceptually valid criteria (Wakefield 1992a, 1992b). With respect to the goal of identifying only individuals with disorders—that is, the goal of avoiding false positives (otherwise known as diagnostic specificity)—conceptual validity is not easy to attain using diagnostic criteria that are framed in terms of symptoms, for the simple reason that the symptoms of many mental disorders can occur as normal responses to certain kinds of environments.

For example, deep sadness can indicate major depressive disorder or it can be a normal reaction to loss. Intense anxiety can be a symptom of generalized anxiety disorder or it can be a normal response to an unusually stressful set of circumstances. Adolescent antisocial behavior can represent a dysfunction such as an inability to empathize with others' needs, an inability to function according to social rules, or an inability to inhibit impulses and thus can indicate a conduct disorder; or such behavior can represent the consequences of a rational decision to join a gang and go along with gang antisocial activities as a way to protect oneself in a dangerous neighborhood. Although excessive alcohol intake is a manifestation of dependence, it can also represent a transient youthful attempt to be exuberantly excessive that involves neither addiction nor abuse. (Some of these examples are developed in "Examples of the False-Positives Problem in DSM-IV-TR.") In these and many other instances, use of criteria based exclusively on symptoms may result in disorder diagnoses of potentially large numbers of nondisorder conditions that have the same "symptoms" as the disorders.

Implications of False Positives in DSM

Concern about possible false positives is not confined to debate among mental health professionals. The criteria for many categories of disorders have been challenged as being overinclusive by lay people in diverse public forums. These disorders include, for example, attention-deficit/hyperactivity disorder, conduct disorder, oppositional defiant disorder, learning disorders, sexual dysfunction, antisocial personality disorder, depression (as opposed to normal unhappiness), paraphilias, gender identity disorder, premenstrual dysphoric disorder, and personality disorder.

There are many reasons why false positives are of concern to the lay public. One reason is worry about excessive medical costs. For example, a common objection to insurance parity for mental disorders has been that mental health professionals do not adequately distinguish normal unhappiness from pathological depression or adjustment disorder, so that treatment for all manner of normal misery becomes reimbursable. Perceptions that criteria are manifestly overinclusive also fuel suspicions that financial self-interest on the part of mental health professionals plays a role in determining normal behavior to be pathological. Other reasons involve broader social issues, such as fear of undermining efforts to achieve social change by placing the causes of problems inside the person; ethical concerns about inappropriate treatments for nondisorder conditions, especially in children; and fear of reducing personal responsibility for one's actions when negative traits or criminal behaviors are labeled as disorders. Further reasons for public concern about false positives are more personal, such as fear of stigma, issues of self-esteem, and the desire to obtain an accurate answer to the question "Is anything wrong with me (or with my child)?"

Potential misdiagnosis of children's and adolescents' conditions is a particularly active area of public concern. Media stories have suggested that some psychiatrically healthy children who are behind in school for various reasons may be considered to have learning disorders and may be routed to special education rather than to other more appropriate and less expensive services. Media stories also express the concern that some normally rambunctious children, responding to excessive constraints in today's classrooms and home environments, may be mislabeled as having attention-deficit/hyperactivity disorder and thus be inappropriately medicated.

Apart from public concern about being falsely labeled as having a mental disorder, the false-positives problem also has implications for the practice of psychiatry. Because DSM is so widely used, the validity or invalidity of its criteria has dramatic implications for the integrity of the entire mental health field. With respect to clinical work, if clinicians mislabel conditions as disorders on the basis of DSM criteria, this may bias them toward conceptualizing problems and selecting treatments in a nonoptimal manner, because of the erroneous assumption that something has gone wrong inside the individual. However, clinical populations are highly self-selected, and clinicians can use their common sense and clinical expertise to adjust for potential flaws in the criteria, so in principle, the danger of false-positive diagnoses can be minimized in clinical settings.

The greater problem stems from the fact that DSM criteria are used in many other contexts and settings (such as research sample selection, general medical practices, courtrooms, and epidemiological studies), where there may be no such corrective mechanisms to make up for deficiencies in the criteria but where false positives can be just as problematic. For example, DSM criteria are often used in sample selection for etiological studies and in treatment outcome trials, and if samples are composed of heterogeneous groups of individuals with disorders and individuals without disorders, the results may be misleading, uninterpretable, and ungeneralizable to a population with disorders. Moreover, real etiological factors and real treatment effects may be obscured. Consider the following example: If, through the use of criteria for major depressive disorder, many people without disorders who are reacting normally to major life losses are classified as having major depressive disorder, treatment trials involving such subjects might yield results that seem to indicate that medication is no more effective than behavioral or cognitive intervention for depression—even if the population without disorders is helped more by medication—because the effect may be obscured by the disproportionate improvement of the group without disorders in response to psychosocial interventions. Moreover, because many normal reactions are self-limiting, the magnitude of the effects of treatment of disorders may be obscured if disorders are not present in a substantial part of the experimental and control samples, and the effect size in comparison with that in the group of control subjects not receiving treatment may appear weaker than it actually is.

Another reason for concern about false positives is that there is currently a strong movement to train general practitioners to diagnose and treat some mental disorders. Such nonpsychiatrically trained medical personnel may rely more heavily on diagnostic criteria, resulting in an increased likelihood of false positives. There are also policy implications: if treatment studies use samples that include many subjects whose conditions are falsely diagnosed as disorders because of invalid criteria, any standard-of-care guidelines based on those outcome studies may be skewed toward the needs of those who do not have disorders. Additionally, the potential implications of invalidity are particularly great for DSM-IV-TR's intended use with community populations in psychiatric epidemiological surveys, which often guide mental health policy and funding decisions. In such studies, because the percentage of subjects without disorders is large, even small false-positive rates can greatly inflate prevalence estimates. The fact that the prevalence estimates yielded by recent epidemiological surveys appear to be implausibly high seems to have undermined confidence in such studies as guides for policy making. For these and other reasons having to do with the long-term credibility of the mental health professions, professionals should be very concerned about the false-positives problem.

Strengths and Weaknesses of the DSM-IV-TR Definition of *Psychiatric Disorder*

In principle, there are two basic sources of overdiagnosis. First, the definition of *mental disorder* that guides the formulation of criteria sets may be inappropriately overinclusive. Second, even if the guiding definition is correct, false positives can occur if the criteria sets for specific disorders do not conform to the requirements of the definition. Thus, to understand the potential sources of false positives in DSM-IV-TR, it is useful to start by examining its definition of *mental disorder:*

> In DSM-IV, each of the mental disorders is conceptualized as a clinically significant behavioral or psychological syndrome or pattern that occurs in an individual and that is associated with present distress (e.g., a painful symptom) or disability (i.e., impairment in one or more important areas of functioning) or with a significantly increased risk of suffering death, pain, disability, or an important loss of freedom. In addition, this syndrome or pattern must not be merely an expectable and culturally sanctioned response to a particular event, for example, the death of a loved one. Whatever its original cause, it must currently be considered a manifestation of a behavioral, psychological, or biological dysfunction in the individual. Neither deviant behavior (e.g., political, religious, or sexual) nor conflicts that are primarily between the individual and society are mental disorders unless the deviance or conflict is a symptom of a dysfunction in the individual, as described above. (American Psychiatric Association 2000, p. xxxi)

One of us (J.C.W.) analyzed and critiqued the DSM definition of *mental disorder* in several articles (Wakefield 1992a, 1992b, 1993, 1996, 1997a), and we will not present that material here. Rather, using that work, we will review a few major strengths and weaknesses of the definition and then propose a revised version.

Regarding strengths, the definition makes four useful points. First, a disorder is something in the individual; it is not simply a bad relationship or poor role performance. Second, the internal condition, whose existence must be inferred from evident symptoms, is a dysfunction; that is, something must have gone wrong with the way that the internal mechanism normally functions (Klein 1978; Spitzer and Endicott 1978). Many problematic internal states, such as ignorance, lack of skill, lack of talent, sadness due to a loss, and foolhardiness, are not disorders in the medical sense because they are not dysfunctions. As noted, in the case of mental disorders, the dysfunctional mechanism must be a cognitive, motivational, behavioral, emotional, or other psychological mechanism. (*Mechanism* is used here without any mechanistic implications about the nature of the mind but simply as the term is commonly used in the evolutionary literature to refer to any inner process or structure.)

Third, a dysfunction of some internal mechanism is not enough to imply a disorder. Many things that go wrong with various mental and physical mechanisms do not merit being called disorders, because they do not have sufficiently negative implications for the individual's overall well-being. The difference between dysfunctions that can be classified as disorders, and dysfunctions that cannot be classified as disorders, thus lies in whether the dysfunction causes significant harm to the person.

Finally, the definition makes clear that the distress or disability must be due to a dysfunction and cannot be due only to social deviance, disapproval by others, or conflict with society or with others. This requirement is meant to preclude the misuse of psychiatry for social control purposes, as occurred in Soviet psychiatry.

The definition has several weaknesses. First, the use of the phrase *clinically significant* is circular in a definition of *disorder*, because the decision about whether a syndrome or pattern is clinically significant depends on whether it is considered a disorder. Second, the list of possible harmful effects, which has grown through successive editions of DSM, has become unwieldy. Clauses have been added to take care of specific problem categories, so the list has an ad hoc quality. There is the sense that it is only a matter of time until yet further clauses are added. Any significant harm directly caused by a dysfunction will make the dysfunction qualify as a disorder.

There are also problems with defining disability as "impaired function." If this includes impaired function of an internal mechanism, it leads to counterexamples; for instance, a specific gene can be impaired and dysfunctional without causing a disorder. There is also a general problem of distinguishing normal variation in ability from pathological disability; for example, the inability to excel at sports is not necessarily a disability. The notion of disability seems to depend on a prior understanding of function and dysfunction (Wakefield 1997b).

The most serious problem, however, is that there is no explanation or analysis of the critical concept of dysfunction. Any definition of *disorder* in terms of the closely related concept of dysfunction is inadequate unless dysfunction undergoes some independent analysis. In lieu of addressing its definition of *dysfunction*, DSM-IV-TR includes a statement apparently intended to reduce the number of false positives—namely, that a disorder cannot be an expectable or socially sanctioned response to events. It is clear, however, that this statement is not a substitute for a definition of *dysfunction*. Many forms of unexpected culturally unsanctioned functioning (e.g., bad manners, petty crime, defiance of social conventions, or civil disobedience based on high moral principles) are not necessarily disorders. Moreover, normal reactions to external stresses (e.g., grief, terror) can be unexpectable and harmful, and nondysfunctional internal conditions such as illiteracy, greediness, or slovenliness can be unexpectable and harmful, yet not disorders. Conversely, some conditions that are dysfunctions can be quite expectable in context, such as posttraumatic stress disorder after a severe trauma. Indeed, most of the V code conditions (conditions included in the DSM-IV-TR chapter titled "Other Conditions That May Be a Focus of Clinical Attention") are not expectable and are harmful but are not disorders. Thus the definition fails to adequately operationally define *dysfunction*.

Although we think that the DSM definition of *disorder* has some limitations, we do not think that the false positives resulting from the use of DSM criteria are due primarily to a faulty definition of *mental disorder*. This is because the strengths of the current definition, and in particular its requirement that there be dysfunction in the individual, would be enough to eliminate most false positives if the criteria sets properly conformed to this definition. Rather, the disparity between the definition and the criteria sets is the source of most false positives (Wakefield 1997a).

Proposed Clarification of the Definition of *Disorder* as "Harmful Dysfunction"

Wakefield (1992a, 1992b, 1993, 1999a, 1999b, 1999c) argued that the concept of disorder, as it applies to both physical and mental conditions, is that of a harmful dysfunction, and a mental disorder would thus be a harmful mental dysfunction. Unlike most standard analyses that claim either that disorder is a value concept or that disorder is a factual scientific concept, this is a hybrid analysis that claims that disorder contains both value ("harm") and scientific or factual ("dysfunction" as failure of a naturally selected function) components. We propose that Wakefield's analysis of disorder be adopted as a guideline for defining *disorder* in DSM-V.

What is a dysfunction according to Wakefield's analysis? A reasonable supposition is that *dysfunction* implies an unfulfilled function of some internal mechanism. But the kinds of functions that are relevant are not those that result from social or personal decisions to use a part of the mind or body in a certain way. For example, although the nose has the function of holding up one's eyeglasses, the fact that one's nose does not do a good job of holding up glasses implies nothing in itself about nasal pathology.

It can be concluded, then, that the only relevant functions are those that are the "natural functions" of some internal mechanism—that is, functions that the mechanism possesses in virtue of how human beings are designed by evolution. Natural functions are not merely the beneficial effects of a mechanism. The language of function is used to indicate that certain effects are so complex, beneficial, and intricately structured that they cannot be accidental side effects of random causal processes but, like the intentionally designed functions of artifacts, must somehow be part of the explanation of why the underlying mechanisms exist and are structured as they are. (Such functions are often said to be what the mechanism is "designed" to do.) Just as it is not a fortunate and amazing accident that pens are so structured that they enable a person to write, and automobiles are so structured that they can transport someone from place to place (these useful effects were in the minds of the designers and manufacturers of such artifacts, and the effects guided the construction of the artifacts), so it cannot be accidental that the eyes see, the hands grasp, one feels fear in the face of danger, or one is thirsty when one needs water. These effects must have somehow played a role in shaping the very mechanisms that have the effects. This intuitive sense of design is at the root of the concepts of function, dysfunction, and disorder. Function attributions implicitly make an unusual explanatory claim—namely, that the underlying mechanism is the way it is partly because of its effects. One can make such inferences without knowing anything about the actual mechanisms. For example, circumstantial evidence suggests that there exist designed mechanisms for producing thought, emotion, sleep, sexual arousal, impulse control, social conscience, and so on, even if it is unknown what these mechanisms are. Indeed, many of DSM's categories (e.g., sleep disorders, sexual and gender identity disorders) clearly correspond to types of inferred designed mechanisms that have gone wrong.

This analysis of function in terms of the explanatory power of effects does not by itself explain how an effect (e.g., pumping, seeing) could explain its own cause (the heart, the eyes), nor does the analysis provide a criterion by which natural functions can be scientifically distinguished from other effects more precisely than by intuition. The analysis inevitably leads one to ask, What kind of underlying process could possibly be responsible for such seeming "design" in natural systems without any designer? To answer this question, one needs a theory about how such explanatory effects can come about (e.g., how the heart's effect of pumping the blood could have shaped the heart or could explain why hearts exist). Earlier accounts of this phenomenon include Aristotle's "final causes" and Aquinas's "God's intentions." The modern answer is that evolutionary theory provides the only plausible scientific account of how the effects of a mechanism can explain the existence and structure of the mechanism. According to evolutionary theory, some effects of a mechanism were beneficial to past organisms and thereby caused the natural selection of the mechanism and thus its existence in present-day organisms. Consequently, those effects are part of an explanation of the existence and structure of the mechanism in present-day organisms. Such naturally selected effects are the natural functions of the respective mechanisms. This theoretical argument leads to the conclusion that disorders are failures of mechanisms to perform functions for which they were naturally selected.

A dysfunction, then, is a failure of an internal mechanism to perform one of the functions for which it is naturally designed. When this definition is applied, ignorance, slipping eyeglasses, and other problematic cases are not considered disorders, because in none of those kinds of cases is there a failure of some mechanism to work as it was designed to work or a failure of a mechanism to perform a function it was designed to perform. In contrast, for example, pumping the blood is a natural function of the heart because it is clear from the nature of the intricate mechanisms involved in the heart's pumping of the blood and the role of pumping in broader vital processes that the pumping cannot be an accidental by-product of having a heart but rather must somehow be part of the explanation of why the heart exists and how it is structured. Consequently, the heart's failure to pump the blood is a dysfunction because it is a failure of the heart to perform one of its natural functions. Such a dysfunction is a disorder because it is a harmful dysfunction.

In sum, a careful analysis of the concept of function (and by implication, dysfunction) leads to the conclusion that the most viable approach is based on the notion of function in terms of what a mechanism is designed to do, where "design" may be grounded in evolutionary theory, in a deistic conception, or in some other theory that implies that some of the mechanism's effects actually shaped the mechanism itself. A natural function is not just any benefit or effect provided by a mechanism; it is only a benefit or effect that explains why the mechanism exists and why it has the form that it does. Such explanations apply equally to physical mechanisms and to mental mechanisms, such as perception, language, learning, action, belief, emotion, thought, and motivation.

Why the Harm Requirement Is Necessary

Those who would like to see the concept of disorder as a purely factual scientific one might be tempted to think that "failure of a naturally designed function" is a sufficient analysis of dysfunction and that disorders are only such dysfunctions. However, both lay and professional behavior regarding classification demonstrates that the concept is more complex and contains a value component. Specifically, unless a dysfunction causes harm, it is not considered a disorder. For example, an inability to learn to read because of a dysfunction in the corpus callosum (assuming that this theory about some forms of dyslexia is correct) is harmful in literate societies but not harmful in preliterate societies, where reading is not a skill that is taught or valued, and thus this inability is not a disorder in those societies. Most people have what physicians call benign anomalies—that is, minor malformations that are the result of genetic or developmental errors but that cause no significant problem—and such anomalies are not considered disorders. If, for example, a malfunction of a gene causes an individual to lack an immune system receptor (this is a clear dysfunction) but the immune system is so redundant that loss of the receptor causes no harm, this condition is not considered a disorder. As a last example, a certain proportion of male sperm are clearly malformed and dysfunctional, but these internal dysfunctions are not considered disorders unless they cause harm in the form of impairment of reproductive function. It is simply not the case that dysfunction by itself constitutes a disorder.

In summary, we believe that the definition of *disorder* as "harmful dysfunction" has several important strengths. First, it is clearly applicable to psychiatric conditions. Second, it appears to capture the same concept of disorder that is used in physical medicine. Third, on the basis of studies of classificatory judgments, the definition appears to reflect a concept widely accepted by mental health professionals and the lay public. Fourth, it appears to possess more power to explain classificatory judgments about disorder and nondisorder than any other available definition.

Most definitions of *disorder* claim either that it is sheerly a value concept or that it is sheerly a factual scientific concept. This is a hybrid analysis that claims that disorder contains both a value component ("harm"), which represents the pragmatic nature of medicine as a profession, in that health care providers are socially sanctioned to intervene in negatively evaluated conditions; and a scientific or factual component ("dysfunction" as failure of a naturally selected function), which represents the specific, objectively defined domain of negative conditions (as opposed to crime, ignorance, poverty, and so on) with which medicine is concerned.

The harmful-dysfunction analysis resolves the ambiguity of the concept of dysfunction in the DSM-IV-TR definition by specifying that *dysfunction* refers to failures of mental mechanisms to perform their naturally selected functions. The use of natural selection offers seemingly the only scientifically objective benchmark for when things go wrong in the medically relevant sense; otherwise, it would appear that disorder becomes solely a value concept. The analysis also resolves the ad hoc nature of the list of harms in the DSM-IV-TR definition by using the generic term *harm* and requiring simply that the dysfunction cause significant harm (judged by social values) if it is to be considered a disorder.

Limitations of the Harmful-Dysfunction Analysis

Critiques have been directed at both the dysfunction and harm requirements of the harmful-dysfunction analysis. With respect to the dysfunction requirement, the major objection has been to the evolutionary aspect of the definition and the epistemological challenges it raises. If dysfunctions are failures of internal mechanisms to perform naturally selected functions, then, given the very limited knowledge of the evolution of mental mechanisms and the difficulty of knowing what factors shaped human brain structures, how can dysfunctions be identified? The harmful-dysfunction analysis does not resolve such epistemological problems; rather, the analysis states what it means to claim that a condition is a disorder. Precisely establishing the nature of the dysfunction is another matter. The analysis provides a framework for pursuing the knowledge needed to make the desired discriminations and for incorporating future knowledge. In addition, there is often circumstantial evidence from which one can judge with some plausibility the functions and dysfunctions of a mechanism (or at least that a function or dysfunction likely exists), with no need for detailed direct knowledge of the evolution of the mechanism. Indeed, practitioners of physical medicine made such judgments for centuries without any understanding of evolution. The fact that the function of the eye is vision—or even, as William Harvey discovered, that the function of the heart is to pump the blood—can be established from complex webs of evidence without evolutionary knowledge. Revealingly, even those who reject evolutionary theory, such as religious fundamentalists, make essentially the same judgments of function and dysfunction based on the effects that a mechanism is designed to have.

Another objection is that when the evolutionary approach is used, almost any negative behavior could be classified as a disorder, because some function could be cited as failing. For example, any type of social deviance could be said to represent a failure of the natural functions responsible for human social interaction. However, the evolutionary view of dysfunction according to the harmful-dysfunction analysis requires that there be a failure of internal mechanisms to operate the way they are evolutionarily designed to operate. There are many normal causal pathways that do not involve dysfunction and that lead to failure to perform a function, and such conditions are not disorders. For example, if the performance of a function is blocked by environmental conditions (e.g., one cannot reproduce because there are no potential partners or only infertile partners around), that is not a dysfunction. Furthermore, if one internal mechanism overrides another and thus leads to failure to perform a function (e.g., a monk's belief system overrides his capacity to talk and leads to failure to engage in the function of speech), that is also not a dysfunction. If social deviance is caused by a reaction to social conditions or lack of nondeviant opportunities, then the deviance is not a disorder (see, for instance, the discussion of conduct disorder in "Examples of the False-Positives Problem in DSM-IV-TR"). Indeed, the harmful-dysfunction analysis has been used to understand the distinction between normal deviance and disorder in the context of adolescent antisocial behavior (Kirk et al. 1999; Wakefield et al. 2002).

With regard to the harm component, one criticism is that the component potentially leads to a radical cultural relativity of disorder because judgments of harm differ based on cultural values. It is true that the harm requirement does lead to a minimal amount of cultural relativity that seems appropriate. The example (presented in "Why the Harm Requirement Is Necessary") of an inability to learn to read in a preliterate society that does not value reading can be used here. A dysfunction of the corpus callosum that limits the ability to learn to read would not constitute a disorder. However, the harmful-dysfunction analysis does not inevitably open the door to radical cultural relativity, because its definition of *disorder* includes both harm and dysfunction. In contrast to harm, dysfunctions are evaluated based on a consideration of species-specific evolutionary function, and thus dysfunction is independent of cultural concepts of normality. For this reason, a culture can actually be wrong about what constitutes a dysfunction, as in societies in which endemic malaria has been considered the normal human state. Consequently, the harmful-dysfunction analysis sets a strict limit on cultural relativity of disorder; each society can influence the range of disorders only by deciding which possible dysfunctions (which are more or less the same cross-culturally) are considered harmful. In essence, cultures can declare certain dysfunctions not to be disorders, but they cannot create a disorder out of the whole cloth of local values. Of course, different societies may have culturally determined erroneous theories of what dysfunctions are, but culture has nothing to do with what are and are not failures of naturally selected functions.

The harm requirement might also be questioned on the grounds that it seems to allow any harm whatever, even trivial harm, to be sufficient for a dysfunction to be a disorder. It is indeed important to recognize that harm is on a continuum and that trivial harm would not make a condition a disorder. There is clearly some threshold of significance or substantialness that the harm must reach to warrant attribution of disorder. The harmful-dysfunction analysis does not address how to set this threshold (a boundary-setting problem); it requires only that there be significant or adequate harm. Indeed, the categorical nature of DSM-IV (and DSM-IV-TR) diagnoses has been criticized more generally for offering no guidance on such boundary issues regarding where to set the threshold.

It could be argued that some disorders, such as antisocial personality disorder, do not harm the individual. On the other hand, by social standards, antisocial personality disorder could be considered to constrain the personality in a way that is harmful in the sense that the individual cannot live what is socially considered a fully desirable life. Or, to account for face validity reactions about antisocial personality disorder and other conditions, one might argue that harm must occur to the individual or others as judged by social standards.

Examples of the False-Positives Problem in DSM-IV-TR

We contend that the main reason for the false-positives problem in DSM-IV-TR is that the diagnostic criteria are often inconsistent with the dysfunction requirement for disorder—that the symptoms be caused by a dysfunction—as put forward not only by the harmful-dysfunction analysis but by the DSM-IV-TR definition of *disorder* as well. We offer here several examples of apparent invalidities in DSM-IV-TR criteria, invalidities that are due to failure to meet the dysfunction requirement:

- The criteria for major depressive disorder contain an exclusion for uncomplicated bereavement (up to 2 months of symptoms after the loss of a loved one is considered normal) but no exclusions for equally normal reactions to other major losses, such as a terminal medical diagnosis in oneself or a loved one, separation from one's spouse, the end of an intense love affair, or loss of one's job and retirement fund. Reactions to such losses may satisfy DSM diagnostic criteria but are not necessarily disorders. If, in grappling with such a loss, one experiences, for example, just 2 weeks of depressed mood, diminished pleasure in usual activities, insomnia, fatigue, and a diminished ability to concentrate on work tasks, one's reaction to the loss satisfies DSM-IV-TR criteria for major depressive disorder, even though such a reaction need not imply pathology any more than it does in bereavement. Clearly, the essential requirement that there be a dysfunction in a depressive disorder—perhaps one in which loss-response mechanisms are not responding proportionately to loss as designed—is not adequately captured by the DSM-IV-TR criteria set.

The "disorder-nondisorder" distinction for depression should not be confused with the traditional "reactive-endogenous" distinction. Endogenous depressions that fulfill the symptom criteria for a major depressive episode certainly are disorders, and some reactive depressions represent proportionate, designed responses to environmental events that do not involve any internal dysfunction and are not disorders. But some reactions to loss can be of such disproportionate intensity or duration that they imply the probability of a breakdown in the designed, adaptive functioning of loss-response mechanisms. Thus, many reactive depressions that meet DSM-IV criteria are indeed disorders, in which the triggering event interacts with inner processes and dispositions to produce a dysfunction. Just as there can be disorder reactions to loss of a loved one, so also there can be disorder reactions to other losses. Among reactive depressions to a variety of losses, some are disorders and some are not, and the problem is that DSM-IV-TR criteria do not adequately distinguish the disorder reactions from the nondisorder reactions.

- Adjustment disorder is defined in terms of a reaction to an identifiable stressor that either 1) causes marked distress that is in excess of what would be expected from exposure to the stressor or 2) significantly impairs academic, occupational, or social functioning. The first, "greater than expected" criterion allows a disorder diagnosis to be made with regard to the top third, say, of the normal distribution of reactivity to stress and so does not adequately deal with normal variation. Moreover, it does not take into account the contextual factors that may provide good reasons for one person to react more intensely than others. The second, "role impairment" criterion classifies as evidence of a disorder even normal reaction to adversity that temporarily impairs functioning (e.g., one does not want to socialize or one does not feel up to going to work). But temporarily retreating from normal role functioning is often exactly how normal coping or adjustment responses work. Here, too, the criteria contain an exclusion for bereavement but not for other equally normal reactions to misfortunes other than death of a loved one. Clearly, the essence of an adjustment disorder is that something has gone wrong with normal coping mechanisms, which are presumably designed to return the individual, gradually and perhaps after a period of retreat, to homeostasis after some stress or change in life circumstances. This essential element of a dysfunction in coping mechanisms is not captured by the DSM-IV-TR criteria set.

- For a DSM-IV-TR diagnosis of substance abuse, which concerns the negative consequences of use, to be made, one of four criteria must be met: poor role performance at work or at home because of substance use; recurrent substance-related legal difficulties; substance use in hazardous circumstances, such as driving under the influence of alcohol; or continued use despite having persistent social or interpersonal problems due to substance use, such as arguments with family members about the consequences of intoxication. These criteria are not valid indicators of disorder and are inconsistent with the DSM-IV-TR definition of *mental disorder*, which asserts that "symptoms" must not be due to conflict with society. Arrests for illegal activity and use of drugs despite disapproval of family members are exactly the kinds of social conflicts that are insufficient for diagnosis of a disorder according to the DSM-IV-TR definition. For example, according to DSM-IV-TR, continuing to use alcohol or drugs despite arguments with one's spouse about alcohol or drug use is sufficient by itself for a diagnosis of substance abuse. Therefore, if you drink or smoke marijuana, your spouse can give you a mental disorder simply by arguing with you about it and can cure you by becoming more tolerant of your being intoxicated! Being arrested more than once for disorderly conduct is also sufficient for diagnosis; therefore, one's diagnostic status depends on the diligence of the local police force. As for the "hazardous use" criterion, it is clear that very large numbers of people drive under the influence of alcohol for all kinds of foolish reasons, and a person need not have a mental disorder to do so.

- The category of acute stress disorder seems to imply that normal-range stress responses are pathological. If a terrible event (such as threat of death, injury, or rape) causes fear, helplessness, or horror (as it typically might), and one has stress-response symptoms (e.g., one feels in a daze and "out of it," thinks about the event, or reacts to reminders of the event in a way that is distressing or impairing) for at least 2 days, one is considered to have a disorder. Moreover, the criteria indicate that the more extreme dissociative symptoms need be present only while one is experiencing the event; they need not continue after the event itself. After the event, according to the criteria, one need only be distressed by reminders of the event or keep processing thoughts about the event, try to avoid those reminders, and remain anxious and continue to have impaired functioning for 2 days. It would seem that after such an event, many normal-range reactions might include such features. There is no doubt that some acute stress responses are so severe and harmful that they are disorders, but the DSM-IV-TR criteria do not adequately distinguish these genuine disorders from intense, normal stress reactions.

- The diagnostic criteria for conduct disorder allow the diagnosis of a disorder to be made in adolescents responding with antisocial behavior to peer pressure, to the dangers of a deprived or threatening environment, or to abuses at home. For example, if a girl who is attempting to avoid escalating sexual abuse by her stepfather lies to her parents about her whereabouts and often stays out late at night despite their prohibitions, and then, tired during the day, often skips school, with the result that her academic functioning becomes impaired, a diagnosis of conduct disorder can be made (criteria 11, 13, and 15). Rebellious children or adolescents, or children or adolescents who fall in with the wrong crowd and who skip school and repetitively shoplift and vandalize, also meet criteria for this diagnosis. However, a paragraph in the "Specific Culture, Age, and Gender Features" section of the DSM-IV-TR text for conduct disorder states that "consistent with the DSM-IV definition of mental disorder, the Conduct Disorder diagnosis should be applied only when the behavior in question is symptomatic of an underlying dysfunction within the individual and not simply a reaction to the immediate social context" (American Psychiatric Association 2000, p. 96) and that "it may be helpful for the clinician to consider the social and economic context in which the undesirable behaviors have occurred" (p. 97). If this paragraph's substance had been incorporated into the diagnostic criteria, many of the false positives could have been eliminated. Unfortunately, in epidemiological studies and research contexts as well as some clinical contexts, the nuances of the text are likely to be ignored.

- Separation anxiety disorder is diagnosed in children on the basis of symptoms that last at least 4 weeks and indicate age-inappropriate, excessive anxiety concerning separation from those to whom the individual is attached. The symptoms (e.g., excessive distress when separation occurs, worry that some event will lead to separation, worry that harm will come to attachment figures, refusal to go to school because of fear of separation, reluctance to be alone or without major attachment figures) are just the sorts of things children experience when they have a normal, intense separation anxiety response. The criteria thus do not provide the user of DSM-IV-TR with any guidance on how to distinguish between a true disorder, in which separation responses are triggered inappropriately, and normal responses to unusual perceived threats to the child's primary bond due to a caregiver's unreliability or other serious disruptions. For example, in a study involving children of military personnel at three bases (Bickman et al. 1995) that happened to take place at the time of Desert Storm, when many parents of the children were in fact leaving for the Middle East, an area where children knew that parents could be killed or injured, the level of separation anxiety was high enough among many of the children that they would qualify as having separation anxiety disorder according to DSM-IV-TR criteria (relative to typical separation responses at their ages, their reactions were "excessive"), but in fact the children were responding with proportional, normal-range separation responses to a highly unusual environment in which they had realistic concerns that parents would not come back (A.M. Brannan, personal communication, March 1996). Psychiatrically healthy children whose attachments are threatened in reality could thus be treated as though they had attachment responses indicative of a disorder, rather than having their real attachment needs addressed.

Limitations of the Clinical Significance Criterion in Eliminating False Positives

The most notable attempt in DSM-IV to make general progress on the false-positives problem is the addition of the following requirement, or a rough equivalent, to about half of the criteria sets in the manual: Symptoms must cause "clinically significant distress or impairment in social, occupational, or other important areas of functioning." The goal of this criterion, which we will call the *clinical significance criterion* (CSC), is to set an impairment or distress threshold for diagnosis so that false positives are eliminated in cases in which there is minimal harm to the individual, and in a few instances the criterion does improve validity. However, requiring "clinically significant" distress or role impairment as a criterion for distinguishing disorder from nondisorder is circular because "clinically significant" in this context can only mean that the impairment is significant enough to imply the existence of a disorder. The phrase offers no real guidance in deciding whether the level of impairment is or is not sufficient to imply disorder.

Furthermore, it does not deal with a large number of potential false positives, specifically those in which there may be harm but no dysfunction (Spitzer and Wakefield 1999). For example, the psychiatrically healthy child in a threatening environment whose aggressive behavior meets the criteria for conduct disorder, and the similarly healthy girl who is threatened by a school bully and whose apparent mutism meets the selective mutism criteria by virtue or her not speaking at school, do experience distress and significant impairment in functioning as part of their normal reactions and so their conditions are not excluded from diagnosis by the CSC. Although motivations can become so intense and rigid that they are pathological, it seems clear that in some cases, such motivations (e.g., not talking to avoid being beaten up by a bully) can be perfectly normal even though impairing of performance and distressful.

Another problem with the CSC is that indiscriminately adding it to criteria sets may result in false-negative misdiagnoses (i.e., failure to diagnose psychiatric disorders that are in fact present), because the criterion includes such specific forms of harm. For example, the CSCs for the sexual dysfunctions in DSM-IV-TR, found in the diagnostic criteria, state that the disturbance causes "marked distress or interpersonal difficulty" or "clinically significant distress or impairment in social, occupational, or other important areas of functioning." However, it is arguable that the symptomatic criteria for a dysfunction such as male erectile disorder or vaginismus constitute a disorder even if the individual is not distressed by it and it causes no interpersonal difficulty. The CSC seems to imply that if a patient can convince himself or herself and his or her partner not to care about a dysfunction, there is no disorder. Similarly, the DSM-IV-TR requirement that a pattern of substance use cause clinically significant impairment or distress before dependence can be diagnosed could yield large numbers of false negatives. It is not uncommon to encounter addicted individuals whose health is threatened by drug use (and who surely have a disorder) but who are not distressed and who can carry on successful role functioning. The proverbial cocaine-addicted successful stockbroker may be an instance, as may be many tobacco users. The problem in many of these cases is that distress and role impairment are not the only kinds of harms that can be caused by dysfunctions. However, in principle, these kinds of problems could be dealt with by simply requiring significant harm.

Perhaps the most problematic aspect of the CSC is that it reflects a misdiagnosis of the main problem underlying false positives and thus a misdirection of effort. The CSC is based on the assumption that the way to ensure that a condition is pathological is to ensure that it causes sufficient distress or impairment in social or role functioning, an assumption at odds with broader diagnostic practice in medicine. Moreover, DSM false positives most often are due not to a failure of symptoms to reach a threshold of harmfulness but to a failure of symptomatic criteria to indicate an underlying dysfunction. Thus, increasing the level of harms such as distress or impairment is not sufficient for distinguishing disorder from nondisorder. There are two good indicators of this failure in DSM-IV-TR itself. The first is that the most obvious potential false positive in the manual—uncomplicated bereavement as distinguished from major depressive disorder—must be dealt with in an additional special exclusion clause and is not eliminated by the CSC that is added to the criteria set, because normal grief can be just as distressful and role impairing as pathological depression, even though it is not caused by a dysfunction. The second indicator is that although the CSC is added to the criteria for conduct disorder, DSM-IV-TR still includes a textual note that children may satisfy the criteria and not have the disorder because their antisocial behavior may not be due to a dysfunction but may be a normal reaction to a problematic environment. Clearly, the CSC does not address the dysfunction problem.

Ways to Address the False-Positives Problem in DSM-V

We now consider, using the harmful-dysfunction analysis to evaluate their strengths and weaknesses, some of the ways other than the CSC that DSM-IV-TR tries to address the false-positives problem. We also offer some suggestions for how the problem might best be dealt with. Although there is no magic bullet to deal with false positives, many useful tools already exist that can be more systematically applied.

The most obvious way that DSM-IV-TR criteria exclude some false positives is through setting high thresholds in diagnostic criteria, such as thresholds involving the number of symptoms required in a syndrome; the specific nature of the individual symptoms in a syndrome; the required severity, intensity, or frequency of the symptoms; and temporal thresholds regarding duration, persistence, and clustering. However, such strategies for reduction of the number of false positives have two disadvantages. First, attempts to reduce the number of false positives through raising the symptomatic threshold for diagnosis can often inadvertently increase the number of false negatives. Second, the effectiveness of this approach is limited by the fact that although more severe symptoms are generally more harmful, it is not always the case that more severe symptoms imply dysfunction. Severe symptoms can occur in normal responses to unusual environmental stressors. Thus, setting high severity and duration thresholds ineffectively addresses the dysfunction problem.

Another strategy, consistent with the statement about unexpectedness in the DSM-IV-TR definition of *disorder*, is to require that the level of the symptoms be statistically unexpectable. The problem with such criteria based on statistical unexpectedness is, first, that being outside the expectable average zone of a distribution does not imply functional failure, because the normal distribution of responses includes the upper end of the distribution; and, second, that statistically unexpectable responses can be normal responses caused either by statistically unexpectable environments or by statistically unexpectable meanings of environmental events for the individual (e.g., unusual importance of a loss) that make the event more stressful than it would be for others.

For example, oppositional defiant disorder is diagnosed when a child displays, during a period of at least 6 months, certain kinds of defiant behavior, such as loss of temper, arguing with adults, refusing to do chores, and swearing, and "the behavior occurs more frequently than is typically observed in individuals of comparable age and developmental level"

(American Psychiatric Association 2000, p. 102). (Note that the "developmental level" requirement was added in DSM-IV to deal with obvious false positives resulting from the DSM-III-R [American Psychiatric Association 1987] criterion that referred only to age.) However, greater-than-typical frequency of such oppositional behaviors may indicate not a disorder but a normal reaction to a stressful, oppressive, or even abusive home environment, or perhaps socialization in an environment where such behaviors are considered more acceptable than usual. Distinguishing such normal reactions that occur with greater-than-typical frequency from dysfunction should be part of the point of diagnosis, but the DSM-IV-TR criteria do not allow for such discrimination. Finally, diagnosis of a reading disorder is allowed if "reading achievement, as measured by individually administered standardized tests of reading accuracy or comprehension, is substantially below that expected" (American Psychiatric Association 2000, p. 53). Yet a child may perform below grade level for a host of reasons other than a reading disorder. (The same problem affects all the categories of learning disorders.) A similar problem with using statistical criteria was noted for the category of adjustment disorders (see "Examples of the False-Positives Problem in DSM-IV-TR").

Another common strategy is to add to the criteria set specific exclusion clauses aimed at known false positives. For example, criteria for selective mutism require that "the failure to speak is not due to a lack of knowledge of, or comfort with, the spoken language required in the social situation" (American Psychiatric Association 2000, p. 127). They also require that "the disturbance is…not limited to the first month of school" (p. 127). These were added to address specific false positives that had become obvious since the publication of DSM-III-R. Similarly, criteria for pyromania state: "The fire setting is not done for monetary gain, as an expression of sociopolitical ideology, to conceal criminal activity, to express anger or vengeance, to improve one's living circumstances" (p. 671).

However, even when improvements with respect to false positives do occur in this manner on an ad hoc, case-by-case basis, they often do not get to the root of the problem. For example, although the exclusions added to the DSM-IV (and DSM-IV-TR) criteria for selective mutism do eliminate some false positives, the criteria are still invalid; for example, they still result in a disorder diagnosis in a girl who does not speak up in school because she is afraid of a bully who accused her of being a teacher's pet and who threatened to beat her up if she said anything. Such lists may be endless, and one must search for an underlying principle that expresses the reason for thinking there is a disorder rather than a nondisorder response to circumstances. The many exclusions in the criteria for pyromania, for example, might be summarized by stating that a disorder does not exist if the setting of fires is done primarily as a contingent instrumental action in pursuit of other goals and not primarily because of an intrinsic desire to set fires.

The criteria for pyromania also happen to illustrate a more promising approach (one that ultimately should be part of the conceptual goals of all criteria sets)—that is, clearly identifying the dysfunctional process. The criteria include the following: "Tension or affective arousal before the act....Fascination with, interest in, curiosity about, or attraction to fire....Pleasure, gratification, or relief when setting fires" (American Psychiatric Association 2000, p. 671). These criteria attempt to identify the essence of the dysfunction (i.e., what has gone wrong), as do the criteria for many of the impulse control disorders, and this is a very effective strategy for eliminating false positives.

In contrast, one of the weakest and most frustrating strategies is to place comments on the potential invalidity of the criteria in the DSM text, thus identifying the potential invalidity without fixing it. For example, the "Differential Diagnosis" section of the DSM-IV-TR text for learning disorders includes the following: "Learning Disorders must be differentiated from **normal variations in academic attainment** and from scholastic difficulties due to **lack of opportunity, poor teaching,** or **cultural factors**" (American Psychiatric Association 2000, p. 51; bold type in original). Cited in the text are potential exclusions in situations in which "English is not the primary language" or in which there is "greater risk of absenteeism due to more frequent illnesses or impoverished or chaotic living environments" (p. 51). These considerations should have been incorporated into the criteria sets themselves, because the criteria for learning disorders are used in many settings—from education to epidemiology—where these important issues raised in the text may not be considered.

A case of identifying the potential invalidity of the criteria without fixing it is also presented in the text for conduct disorder: "Concerns have been raised that the Conduct Disorder diagnosis may at times be misapplied to individuals in settings where patterns of undesirable behavior are sometimes viewed as protective (e.g., threatening, impoverished, high-crime). Consistent with the DSM-IV definition of mental disorder, the Conduct Disorder diagnosis should be applied only when the behavior in question is symptomatic of an underlying dysfunction within the individual and not simply a reaction to the immediate social context" (American Psychiatric Association 2000, p. 96). In effect, the text of DSM-IV-TR says that the criteria presented for conduct disorder are potentially invalid and subject to false positives. Yet it is the criteria, and not the text, that are used by researchers to identify samples for research and treatment outcome studies and by epidemiologists to establish the extent of the population with disorders.

A more promising strategy is to add modifiers to symptomatic criteria that indicate how disproportionate a response is to environmental triggers. For example, the criteria for body dysmorphic disorder deal with a potentially vast number of false positives—because of the very common but often quite painful concerns that people generally have about imperfections in their appearance—by requiring that the person's concern be "markedly excessive" if a slight physical anomaly is present. This sort of approach, which places the symptom into the situational context and evaluates whether it is a proportionate response, is potentially one of the most effective strategies for addressing the false-positives problem.

However, in most instances, this strategy is not applied effectively. For example, the criteria for specific phobia require that there be "marked and persistent fear that is excessive or unreasonable" (American Psychiatric Association 2000, p. 449), the criteria for generalized anxiety disorder require that "excessive anxiety and worry" be present, and the criteria for separation anxiety disorder require that the individual experience "developmentally inappropriate and excessive anxiety concerning separation." The problem here is that by itself, *excessive* is too vague; one wants to ask, "Excessive relative to what?" And *unreasonable* is potentially problematic because not all mechanisms in the body are designed to operate by reason. For example, regarding phobias, one may be evolutionarily prepared to be afraid of all snakes, even though it is unreasonable to be afraid of the ones that are nonpoisonous. But adding modifiers to symptomatic criteria does have the virtue of attempting to place the symptom in a broader context.

Another way of placing symptoms in a broader context is first to specify the circumstances under which one would expect a normal response and then to define *pathology* as the failure of the response despite the occurrence of the specified circumstances. For example, the criteria for male orgasmic disorder (formerly called inhibited male orgasm) specify that the symptoms persist even when the contextual conditions that are designed to produce a normal male orgasmic response are present: "Persistent or recurrent delay in, or absence of, orgasm following a normal sexual excitement phase during sexual activity that the clinician, taking into account the person's age, judges to be adequate in focus, intensity, and duration" (American Psychiatric Association 2000, p. 552). Such placing of symptoms in context offers the best hope for increasing the validity of criteria sets and eliminating false positives to the degree that operationalized criteria for theoretical constructs are able.

There are many strands to the solution of the false positives problem, but our discussion of criteria suggests that one approach stands out. When symptom criteria are insufficient, disorder and nondisorder can often be distinguished by examining the relationship between context and symptoms. For example, sadness roughly proportional in intensity and duration to recent loss is generally not a disorder, whereas sadness not properly related to loss is likely to be. A dysfunction exists when a person's internal mechanisms are not able to function in the range of environments to which they were designed to respond. Thus, one can construct a test for dysfunction by specifying an environment in which the function is designed to manifest itself; if the function is not manifested in that environment, there is likely a dysfunction. The DSM-IV-TR criteria for male orgasmic disorder offer a good example of this strategy; they specify the conditions under which an orgasmic response is to be expected and specify that there is a disorder only if there is no response under those circumstances. Conversely, in some cases, a response that occurs without appropriate eliciting stimuli may indicate a dysfunction. For example, major depressive disorder may be distinguished from normal sadness by the fact that the emotional response is substantially out of proportion to any experienced loss. Thus, a diagnosis would not be appropriate if the response were a proportionate response to a loss. The criteria for body dysmorphic disorder that were discussed earlier in this section also used this strategy of bringing in the relation between a response and its context to determine if there is a dysfunction; the criteria made clear that even if there is indeed a real defect in appearance, there can still be a disorder if the response is substantially out of proportion to the nature of the problem.

Suggestions for Implementation

What, then, should be done to seriously address the problem of false positives? There are two sources of false positives: the definition of *mental disorder* that guides inclusion decisions may be flawed, and the construction of criteria sets for specific disorders may not satisfy the requirements laid down by the definition of *disorder*. The first problem will be addressed if the harmful-dysfunction analysis or at least its most essential insights are used to reformulate the DSM-IV-TR definition of *mental disorder*.

The second concern will be addressed if each criteria set for each specific disorder is conceptually analyzed to establish whether it meets, to the extent possible, the requirements of the harmful-dysfunction analysis. That is, each criteria set should clearly identify conditions that are harmful and that are caused by an internal dysfunction. When a criteria set does not satisfy these minimal conceptual requirements—and we have shown that many criteria sets do not—it should be modified to be made consistent with the definition. Where possible, the criteria set should identify exactly what is supposed to be going wrong when the specific disorder exists. Of course, incorporated into the criteria should be symptoms that as specifically as possible indicate dysfunction, whether through the number, the severity, the duration, the course, the nature, or other features of the symptoms; in the future, laboratory tests and other kinds of criteria might be added. But adding to symptomatic criteria will not be enough, as we have shown. New strategies need to be tried to improve descriptive criteria during the wait for breakthroughs in etiological theory. In particular, new exclusion clauses should be added, where appropriate, to eliminate from diagnosis normal proportional reactions to circumstances and context. Finally, it should be kept in mind that no algorithmic system is perfect; sufficient flexibility or escape clauses (analogous to current subthreshold diagnoses and not-otherwise-specified categories that allow for diagnosis of what would otherwise be false negatives) must be built into the diagnostic criteria to allow clinicians to exclude false positives, even if conditions satisfy DSM criteria. There is currently no explicit provision for the clinician to override the criteria in cases of false positives.

These suggestions should be implemented in such a way that a structure exists that ensures that the false-positives problem will be taken seriously in the revision process leading up to DSM-V. The apparent extent of the problem across many diagnostic categories makes it clear that there is a need for a committee devoted to ensuring uniform application of these principles across criteria sets. Moreover, there should be a mechanism for identifying and addressing, during the revision process, public concerns about false positives; active engagement with any public or internal criticisms about false positives will go a long way toward reducing criticism. The committee's approach should involve active generation of possible counterexamples to criteria sets by conceptually talented critics in order to test whether the criteria are valid—a bit like a company hiring hackers to try to break into its own computers to see if security is sufficient. When false positives are identified, the chapter titled (in DSM-IV and DSM-IV-TR) "Other Conditions That May Be a Focus of Clinical Attention" must be expanded to accommodate them. Most importantly, there must be the beginnings of an attempt to study and identify the size of the problem empirically—for example, by incorporating scales to detect possible false positives into standard instruments used in clinical trials and epidemiological studies.

In conclusion, we noted in the section "False-Positives Problem in DSM" that DSM-III broke new conceptual ground in the attempt to deal seriously with the public challenge of the antipsychiatry movement. The process leading up to DSM-V offers an opportunity for psychiatry to be equally bold in breaking with past conceptual limits and discharging its responsibility to construct diagnostic criteria that validly distinguish disorders from nondisorders.

References

American Psychiatric Association: Diagnostic and Statistical Manual: Mental Disorders. Washington, DC, American Psychiatric Association, 1952

American Psychiatric Association: Diagnostic and Statistical Manual of Mental Disorders, 2nd Edition. Washington, DC, American Psychiatric Association, 1968

American Psychiatric Association: Diagnostic and Statistical Manual of Mental Disorders, 3rd Edition. Washington, DC, American Psychiatric Association, 1980

American Psychiatric Association: Diagnostic and Statistical Manual of Mental Disorders, 3rd Edition, Revised. Washington, DC, American Psychiatric Association, 1987

American Psychiatric Association: Diagnostic and Statistical Manual of Mental Disorders, 4th Edition. Washington, DC, American Psychiatric Association, 1994

American Psychiatric Association: Diagnostic and Statistical Manual of Mental Disorders, 4th Edition, Text Revision. Washington, DC, American Psychiatric Association, 2000

Ausubel DP: Personality disorder is disease. Am Psychol 16:59–74, 1971

Bickman L, Guthrie PR, Foster EM, et al: Evaluating Managed Mental Health Services: The Fort Bragg Experiment. New York, Plenum, 1995

Foucault M: Madness and Civilization: A History of Insanity in the Age of Reason. Translated by Howard R. New York, Pantheon, 1965

Foucault M: History of Sexuality, Vol 1: An Introduction. New York, Pantheon, 1978

Frances AJ, Widiger TA, Sabshin M: Psychiatric diagnosis and normality, in The Diversity of Normal Behavior: Further Contributions to Normatology. Edited by Offer D, Sabshin M. New York, Basic Books, 1992, pp 3–38

Kendell RE: The concept of disease and its implications for psychiatry. Br J Psychiatry 127:305–315, 1975

Kendell RE: What are mental disorders? in Issues in Psychiatric Classification: Science, Practice, and Social Policy. Edited by Freedman AM, Brotman R, Silverman I, et al. New York, Human Sciences Press, 1986, pp 23–45

King L: What is disease? in Concepts of Health and Disease: Interdisciplinary Perspectives. Edited by Caplan AL, Engelhardt HT Jr, McCartney JJ. Reading, MA, Addison-Wesley, 1981, pp 107–108

Kirk SA, Wakefield JC, Hsieh D, et al: Social context and social workers' judgment of mental disorder. Social Service Review 73:82–104, 1999

Kirmayer LJ, Young A: Culture and context in the evolutionary concept of mental disorder. J Abnorm Psychol 108:446–452, 1999

Klein DF: A proposed definition of mental illness, in Critical Issues in Psychiatric Diagnosis. Edited by Spitzer RL, Klein DF. New York, Raven, 1978, pp 41–71

Laing RD: The Politics of Experience. London, Penguin Books, 1967

Lilienfeld SO, Marino L: Mental disorder as a Roschian concept: a critique of Wakefield's "harmful dysfunction" analysis. J Abnorm Psychol 104:411–420, 1995

Lilienfeld SO, Marino L: Essentialism revisited: evolutionary theory and the concept of disorder. J Abnorm Psychol 108:400–411, 1999

Moore MS: Discussion of the Spitzer-Endicott and Klein proposed definitions of mental disorder (illness), in Critical Issues in Psychiatric Diagnosis. Edited by Spitzer RL, Klein DF. New York, Raven, 1978, pp 85–104

Pichot P: Comment, in Issues in Psychiatric Classification: Science, Practice, and Policy. Edited by Freedman AM, Brotman R, Silverman I, et al. New York, Human Sciences Press, 1986, p 56

Sarbin T: On the futility of the proposition that some people be labeled "mentally ill." J Consult Psychol 31:447–453, 1967

Scadding JG: Diagnosis: the clinician and the computer. Lancet 2:877–882, 1967

Scadding JG: The semantic problem of psychiatry. Psychol Med 20:243–248, 1990

Scheff TJ: Being Mentally Ill: A Sociological Theory. Chicago, IL, Aldine, 1966

Scheff TJ (ed): Labeling Madness. Englewood Cliffs, NJ, Prentice-Hall, 1975

Sedgwick P: Illness—mental and otherwise. Stud Hastings Cent 3:19–40, 1973

Sedgwick P: Psycho Politics. New York, Harper & Row, 1982

Spitzer RL, Endicott J: Medical and mental disorder: proposed definition and criteria, in Critical Issues in Psychiatric Diagnosis. Edited by Spitzer RL, Klein DF. New York, Raven, 1978, pp 15–39

Spitzer RL, Wakefield JC: DSM-IV diagnostic criterion for clinical significance: does it help solve the false positives problem? Am J Psychiatry 156:1856–1864, 1999

Szasz TS: The Myth of Mental Illness: Foundations of a Theory of Personal Conduct, Revised Edition. New York, Harper & Row, 1974

Taylor FK: A logical analysis of the medico-psychological concept of disease. Psychol Med 1:356–364, 1971

Taylor FK: The medical model of the disease concept. Br J Psychiatry 128:588–594, 1976

Wakefield JC: The concept of mental disorder: on the boundary between biological facts and social values. Am Psychol 47:373–388, 1992a

Wakefield JC: Disorder as harmful dysfunction: a conceptual critique of DSM-III-R's definition of mental disorder. Psychol Rev 99:232–247, 1992b

Wakefield JC: Limits of operationalization: a critique of Spitzer and Endicott's (1978) proposed operational criteria for mental disorder. J Abnorm Psychol 102:160–172, 1993

Wakefield JC: DSM-IV: are we making diagnostic progress? Contemporary Psychology 41:646–652, 1996

Wakefield JC: Diagnosing DSM-IV, part 1: DSM-IV and the concept of mental disorder. Behav Res Ther 35:633–650, 1997a

Wakefield JC: Normal inability versus pathological disability: why Ossorio's (1985) definition of mental disorder is not sufficient. Clinical Psychology: Science and Practice 4:249–258, 1997b

Wakefield JC: The concept of mental disorder as a foundation for the DSM's theory-neutral nosology: response to Follette and Houts, part 2. Behav Res Ther 37:1001–1027, 1999a

Wakefield JC: Disorder as a black box essentialist concept. J Abnorm Psychol 108:465–472, 1999b

Wakefield JC: Evolutionary versus prototype analyses of the concept of disorder. J Abnorm Psychol 108:374–399, 1999c

Wakefield JC, Pottick KJ, Kirk SA: Should the DSM-IV diagnostic criteria for conduct disorder consider social context? Am J Psychiatry 159:380–386, 2002

World Health Organization: International Classification of Diseases, 9th Revision, Clinical Modification. Ann Arbor, MI, Commission on Professional and Hospital Activities, 1978

World Health Organization: International Statistical Classification of Diseases and Related Health Problems, 10th Revision, Vol 1. Geneva, World Health Organization, 1992

CHAPTER 3

Should the DSM Diagnostic Groupings Be Changed?

Katharine A. Phillips, M.D., Lawrence H. Price, M.D.,
Benjamin D. Greenberg, M.D., Ph.D.,
Steven A. Rasmussen, M.D.

In this chapter, we wrestle with a diagnostic dilemma that might delight the nosologist but strike many clinicians as theoretical, arcane, and clinically irrelevant: How should DSM disorders be organized? Is the current grouping optimal, or should some disorders be rearranged to more accurately reflect their relationship to one another? We hope to convince the reader that this issue, although it involves theory, is clinically important. This question also provides a window on the radical changes that are likely to occur in future editions of DSM.

The following case exemplifies the clinical relevance of this diagnostic dilemma:

> Ms. A, a 34-year-old, single white woman presented with a chief complaint of "I'm obsessed, and I have lots of compulsive behaviors." Since age 15, she had been preoccupied with her nose, which she thought was "huge, hideous, and horrendous looking." Because of this concern, she sometimes missed school, avoided friends, and felt suicidal. She stated that at times, she realized that her view of her appearance was "probably distorted," but at other times, especially when she was around other people, she was "absolutely, 100% convinced" that her belief was correct. Ms. A was also excessively concerned about germs. She washed her hands up to 50 times a day and avoided activities that she thought might lead to contamination. In addition, she reported a history of hair pulling, which in her 20s had resulted in noticeable hair loss. The patient's family history was notable for Tourette's disorder in a brother.

According to DSM-IV-TR (American Psychiatric Association 2000), Ms. A's obsessions and compulsive behaviors warrant several diagnoses from different sections of the manual: 1) body dysmorphic disorder (BDD), a somatoform disorder; 2) delusional disorder, a psychotic disorder; 3) obsessive-compulsive disorder (OCD), an anxiety disorder; and 4) trichotillomania, an impulse-control disorder. Does Ms. A really have four different disorders from four different diagnostic classes? Or are these obsessions and compulsions symptoms of related disorders? And what are the treatment implications of these different possibilities?

In this chapter, we discuss the following four diagnostic dilemmas, which exemplify the larger question of whether the DSM-IV-TR diagnostic groupings should be changed:

1. Should DSM include a section of "obsessive-compulsive spectrum disorders"? Ms. A's four diagnoses could be conceptualized as members of this hypothesized family of related disorders, a grouping not currently present in DSM-IV-TR.
2. Should the grouping of somatoform disorders be eliminated and the disorders moved to various sections of DSM? Is this section of disorders clinically useful or misleading?
3. Should delusional and nondelusional forms of disorders be merged? Several disorders (e.g., BDD, OCD, and hypochondriasis) have delusional and nondelusional variants that are classified as separate disorders in DSM-IV-TR. For example, Ms. A's preoccupation with her nose would be diagnosed at times as a somatoform disorder (BDD) and at other times as a psychotic disorder (delusional disorder). Should the delusional and nondelusional variants of these disorders be combined to form a single disorder spanning a spectrum of insight?
4. Should DSM include a section of "stress-related disorders"? Should disorders occurring in response to stressful events (such as posttraumatic stress disorder [PTSD] and adjustment disorder) be classified together in a new section to highlight the presumed importance of stress as an etiological factor?

Organizational diagnostic dilemmas in DSM are not limited to these examples. Another example is whether "near-neighbor" Axis I and Axis II disorders (e.g., schizophrenia and schizotypal personality disorder, or social phobia and avoidant personality disorder) should be classified together. Is schizoaffective disorder best classified with the psychotic disorders or the mood disorders?

In this chapter, we first briefly review the organization of DSM-IV-TR and suggest an alternative approach. We then discuss the four diagnostic dilemmas just described, which were debated during the development of DSM-IV (American Psychiatric Association 1994) but not resolved. We discuss research needed to solve these and other organizational diagnostic dilemmas, and we outline some of the challenges and pitfalls that radical reorganization of DSM diagnostic groupings might involve. We end by discussing possible solutions to the overall organizational diagnostic dilemma.

DSM-IV-TR Categories

DSM-IV-TR diagnoses are grouped into 16 categories:

1. Disorders usually first diagnosed in infancy, childhood, or adolescence
2. Delirium, dementia, and amnestic and other cognitive disorders
3. Mental disorders due to a general medical condition
4. Substance-related disorders
5. Schizophrenia and other psychotic disorders
6. Mood disorders
7. Anxiety disorders
8. Somatoform disorders
9. Factitious disorders
10. Dissociative disorders
11. Sexual and gender identity disorders
12. Eating disorders
13. Sleep disorders
14. Impulse-control disorders not elsewhere classified
15. Adjustment disorders
16. Personality disorders

DSM-I (American Psychiatric Association 1952) had only 3 superordinate categories, and DSM-II (American Psychiatric Association 1968) had 10. In DSM-III (American Psychiatric Association 1980), the number of categories was increased to 16, reflecting the diagnostic classes proposed by Washington University investigators. The DSM-III metamorphosis was accomplished primarily by dividing the DSM-II psychosis category into psychotic disorders and affective disorders and by dispersing what were previously termed *neuroses* into the anxiety, somatoform, dissociative, and affective disorder categories. These diagnostic classes were subsequently used, with minor modifications, in DSM-III-R (American Psychiatric Association 1987) and DSM-IV.

In more recent versions of DSM, the guiding principle for the creation of these higher-order classes was descriptive and pragmatic, based on clinical utility and the facilitation of differential diagnosis rather than on an empirical foundation or theory about pathogenesis (Clark et al. 1995; Morey 1991; R.S. Spitzer and Williams 1980; Sullivan and Kendler 1998). Inclusion of each diagnostic class (e.g., anxiety disorders) was based on the "best judgment of the Task Force and its Advisory Committees that such subdivision will be useful" (American Psychiatric Association 1980, p. 7).

Psychiatry's Syndrome-Based Classification System: Stepping-Stone to an Etiologically Based System?

Grouping disorders on the basis of shared clinical features, as was largely done in DSM-IV, is only one of several ways of defining and organizing disorders. Disorders can be described on multiple levels: a symptomatic level, based on a single symptom; a syndromal level, based on a cluster of signs and/or symptoms; a pathophysiological level, based on knowledge of physiological disturbance; and a pathoetiological level, based on knowledge of the causative agents (Preskorn 1995). The following example from nonpsychiatric medicine illustrates this concept: chest pain due to atherosclerotic cardiovascular disease would be described at the symptomatic level as chest pain, at the syndromal level as angina, at the pathophysiological level as myocardial ischemia, and at the pathoetiological level as coronary artery atherosclerosis (although this last level could be taken further, to include causes of atherosclerosis).

Over the years, syndrome-based classification systems in nonpsychiatric medicine have largely been replaced by systems based on pathogenesis (e.g., infectious organisms) (Kendell 1991). It has been argued that classifications based on the structural or functional abnormalities underlying the syndrome are usually more useful and valid (Kendell 1989). Psychiatry has lagged behind other medical specialties in that psychopathology, and the groupings of disorders, is still largely defined at the syndromal level rather than the pathophysiological or etiological level (Compton and Guze 1995). There are several exceptions to this, one of which is the category of mental disorders due to a general medical condition. Another exception is dementia; the disorders in the dementia section share a symptom presentation but are differentiated on the basis of etiology (e.g., dementia due to head trauma, substance-induced persisting dementia).

The fact that DSM is largely free of implications about etiology and pathophysiology is due in part to a lack of knowledge of etiopathology and the contentious nature of etiological assumptions (Kendell 1984). As etiology and pathophysiology become known, they would become the basis of an optimal classification system and optimal diagnostic groupings. This idea is not new. Throughout history, proposals for etiologically based systems—ranging from phrenology to psychoanalytic theory—have alternated with proposals for description-based systems (Frances et al. 1995; Mack et al. 1994). Several millennia ago, for example, Hippocrates believed that mental health depended on the balance of blood, phlegm, black bile, and yellow bile (Frances et al. 1995). In the sixteenth century, Paracelsus developed a classification system for mental disorders that was based on etiology: *vesania* (disorders caused by poison), lunacy (a periodic condition influenced by the phases of the moon), and insanity (diseases caused by heredity) (Frances et al. 1990). In the 1800s, an attempt was made to classify mental illness according to the presence of brain lesions (Mack et al. 1994). Kraepelin hoped that one day there would be an etiologically based system to complement his descriptive one (Mack et al. 1994). More recently, this idea was implied by Robins and Guze (1970) when they noted that a fully validated classification system would require information from laboratory studies.

An etiological approach to classification would have many advantages, including increased validity and accuracy of the classification system. This increase in validity and accuracy would be accomplished by ensuring that phenomenologically similar but etiologically distinct syndromes were not classified together and by improving the ability to identify, treat, and prevent disorders. For example, related disorders would be expected to cluster together in families, which would alert clinicians to screen patients carefully for disorders related to those occurring in family members (e.g., to look for OCD in a patient whose parent had hypochondriasis). Perhaps most importantly, an etiologically based classification scheme would lead to more effective treatments. It is clearly more advantageous to classify fever on the basis of the identity of the infectious organism or other etiological agent than by the presenting clinical feature of pyrexia. Just as penicillin is more effective for fever due to a streptococcal infection than to a neoplasm, one type of antidepressant might in theory prove more effective than another for a type of depression with a particular etiology. Classification should ultimately reflect disease processes.

The current syndrome-based classification system has nonetheless served the field of psychiatry well—for example, by increasing diagnostic reliability, providing a common language and thereby facilitating communication among clinicians, and guiding treatment. However, this system also has notable limitations. It is likely, for instance, that unrelated disorders are grouped together, which falsely implies that there is a meaningful relationship among them. One prospective study found that the anxiety disorders do not appear to constitute a cohesive nosological category; in the study, although panic disorder and phobia shared important etiological factors, generalized anxiety disorder was more closely related etiologically to major depression (Kendler et al. 1995). In another study, although certain syndromes clustered together in a manner similar to the way DSM-III-R groups them (e.g., alcoholism and nicotine dependence), the clustering of other disorders resembled DSM-III-R groupings to only a modest extent (e.g., generalized anxiety disorder and major depression were in the same latent, superordinate class) (Sullivan and Kendler 1998). Some genetic studies of bipolar disorder have found linkage in the same chromosomal regions implicated in schizophrenia, and vice versa (Knowles et al. 1999).

The current syndrome-based classification is best conceptualized as a useful stepping-stone to a more definitive and even more useful classification system. Whether a classification system based on pathogenesis will be simpler or more complex than the current system is unclear. The system would be simpler if different psychiatric disorders are shown to have a common etiological basis, as was the case for scurvy: what appeared to be a variety of "sea diseases," such as putrid gums and spots, were actually due to a common underlying abnormality (Hudson and Pope 1990). However, this approach could alternatively increase the number of diagnoses and superordinate groupings, just as the clinical diagnosis of pneumonia has expanded into scores of etiologically specific diagnoses (Todd and Reich 1989).

With the remarkable advances occurring in molecular genetics, neuroimaging, and other branches of the neurosciences, psychiatry is at the threshold of a new era. Such information will greatly increase understanding of the pathogenesis of psychiatric illness and will substantially inform— even radically change—psychiatry's classification system (Rauch 1996). We anticipate that this new knowledge will greatly inform ongoing debates about psychiatric classification, including the four classification dilemmas discussed in the next section.

Organizational Dilemmas

Should DSM Include a Group of Obsessive-Compulsive Spectrum Disorders?

During the planning of DSM-IV, consideration was given to moving BDD (Phillips and Hollander 1996) and hypochondriasis (Foa et al. 1996) to the anxiety disorders section because of their apparent similarities with OCD. What we consider here is a related concept: should a new section of OCD-like disorders ("obsessive-compulsive spectrum disorders") be included in future editions of DSM? The obsessive-compulsive spectrum concept is an example of how disorders might be reorganized on the basis of a presumably shared pathogenesis. Disorders are posited to have "spectrum membership" on the basis of their similarities with OCD in a variety of domains (see Table 3–1)—not only symptoms, sex ratio, age at onset, course, comorbidity (among disorders within and outside of the spectrum), joint familial loading, and treatment response, but also presumed etiology (Klein 1993). The obsessive-compulsive spectrum shares similarities with some other proposed spectra, such as the schizophrenia spectrum (Faraone et al. 1995) and the affective spectrum (Hudson and Pope 1990), in that membership moves beyond description and is based on the idea that certain disorders have a common pathogenesis.

Because the etiology of OCD and the putative spectrum disorders is not yet known, membership in this family has been based largely on the other criteria just noted. Disorders commonly included in the spectrum are Tourette's disorder, BDD, hypochondriasis, and some of the impulse-control disorders, such as trichotillomania and kleptomania (Hollander and Phillips 1993). These obsessive-compulsive spectrum disorders are widely scattered throughout DSM-IV-TR. Some conceptualizations of the spectrum are quite broad and include a far wider range of disorders, some of which appear quite dissimilar from OCD, such as depersonalization disorder and borderline personality disorder (Hollander and Phillips 1993).

Evidence supporting this theory has been reviewed elsewhere and consists of data from multiple sources (Hollander and Phillips 1993; McElroy et al. 1994). From a descriptive perspective, this theory has considerable face validity, especially for narrower conceptualizations of the spectrum. Many obsessive-compulsive spectrum disorders are characterized primarily by prominent and recurrent intrusive thoughts and/or repetitive behaviors. In addition, spectrum disorders commonly co-occur in clinical settings. For example, approximately 30% of patients with BDD have lifetime OCD (Phillips et al. 1994), whereas more than 20% of patients with Tourette's disorder have lifetime OCD (and more than 40% report a history of subsyndromal obsessive-compulsive symptoms [Leckman et al. 1994]). These figures suggest that these disorders are related, or even symptoms of the same underlying disorder. (On the other hand, BDD is also highly comorbid with major depression, suggesting that BDD may be related to mood disorders [Phillips et al. 1995]).

Family studies support some, but not all, hypothesized relationships among various obsessive-compulsive spectrum disorders. A controlled and blinded family study found that BDD, and either BDD or hypochondriasis, occurred significantly more frequently in first-degree relatives of probands with OCD than in first-degree relatives of control probands, but other putative spectrum disorders (eating disorders or impulse-control disorders) did not (Bienvenu et al. 2000), which suggests that a narrower conceptualization of the spectrum may be more valid than a broader one. Disorders

TABLE 3–1. Similarities between OCD and "obsessive-compulsive spectrum disorders" in selected domains

Domain	Tourette's disorder	BDD	Hypochondriasis	Trichotillomania
Symptoms	++	+++	++	++
Comorbidity with OCD	+++	+++	+	+
Familial relationship	+++	++	+	+
Treatment response	0	++	+/?	+

Note. BDD=body dysmorphic disorder; OCD=obsessive-compulsive disorder.

are also posited to belong to the obsessive-compulsive spectrum on the basis of selective response to serotonin reuptake inhibitors. Although limited data suggest that certain spectrum disorders, such as BDD, do appear to respond preferentially to serotonin reuptake inhibitors (Hollander et al. 1999), the treatment response of most spectrum disorders has been insufficiently studied. The fact that Tourette's disorder responds to antipsychotics, and that disorders such as premenstrual dysphoric disorder (Pearlstein et al. 1997) may respond preferentially to serotonin reuptake inhibitors, illustrates the hazards of using treatment response as the primary determinant of obsessive-compulsive spectrum membership.

Interpreting neurobiological findings with respect to the obsessive-compulsive spectrum concept is particularly problematic. A growing body of research has documented structural abnormalities in the caudate nucleus, and increased activity in the orbitofrontal cortex and caudate nucleus, in patients with OCD (Rauch and Baxter 1998). In contrast, Tourette's disorder and trichotillomania have been associated with structural changes in the putamen and globus pallidus (Rauch and Savage 2000). These findings seem somewhat disparate but can be accommodated by overarching theories of corticostriatal circuitry dysfunction (Rauch and Savage 2000). Neurochemical and neuroendocrine findings in patients with OCD have been weaker and less consistent (Price et al. 1995), and such aspects have generally been understudied in other obsessive-compulsive spectrum conditions, with some notable exceptions (Marazziti et al. 1999). Although research on the neurobiology of putative obsessive-compulsive spectrum disorders is increasing (Stein 2000), the number of studies conducted is still very small, and until more systematic studies are done, neurobiological support for the obsessive-compulsive spectrum will remain severely limited.

The obsessive-compulsive spectrum hypothesis is appealing because it links apparently related disorders. It also moves the current, description-based diagnostic system toward one based on presumed pathogenesis, in which meaningful relationships among disorders are reflected by the organization of those disorders. At present, however, the obsessive-compulsive spectrum concept has important limitations. One is that some of these disorders have undergone little investigation (Rasmussen 1994), even at the syndromal level, and few studies have examined their relationship in direct comparison studies. Data from other studies (e.g., family studies, treatment studies, follow-up studies) are also quite scarce for many of the disorders. Furthermore, some of the putative spectrum disorders have notable similarities with disorders excluded from the spectrum. For example, family history and comorbidity studies support a relationship between hypochondriasis and somatization disorder (Noyes et al. 1994, 1997). Perhaps most importantly, many of the proposed obsessive-compulsive spectrum disorders (Tourette's disorder is an exception) have undergone little neurobiological investigation, the approach with the greatest potential for resolving the spectrum dilemma.

An additional problem is that the obsessive-compulsive spectrum concept itself lacks precision and is poorly operationalized. Criteria for membership are unclear. To be included in the spectrum, how similar must a disorder be to OCD in each domain, and in how many domains must similarities exist? In our view, the lack of operationalized criteria has led to overinclusiveness; some putative obsessive-compulsive spectrum disorders (e.g., borderline personality disorder) appear strikingly dissimilar from OCD (Rasmussen 1994). An additional problem is that OCD itself is likely to be heterogeneous, comprising a number of entities with a somewhat distinct pathogenesis (Rasmussen 1994). For example, Tourette's disorder and trichotillomania may be more similar to a putative "incompleteness" subtype of OCD, whereas BDD and hypochondriasis may be more similar to a putative "harm avoidance" OCD subtype (Richter et al. 1996). Pediatric autoimmune neuropsychiatric disorders associated with streptococcal infections (PANDAS; Swedo et al. 1997) might represent an OCD subtype with a pathophysiology and etiology that differ from those of other forms of OCD. The putative obsessive-compulsive spectrum disorders are also likely to be heterogeneous. Whereas some forms of BDD, for example, appear to overlap with OCD, other forms appear to overlap with eating disorders. The heterogeneity problem does not invalidate the spectrum hypothesis, but it does complicate it.

The obsessive-compulsive spectrum hypothesis offers both promises and pitfalls. It has heuristic and practical clinical utility (e.g., treatment implications) and considerable face validity but only limited empirical support. Because of the paucity of research on many of the putative spectrum disorders, it would be premature to include this grouping of disorders in DSM at this time. Most importantly, data on the pathogenesis of these disorders are lacking. Nonetheless, it is likely that future research will reveal that the pathogenesis of some—but not all—of these disorders overlaps, and it is likely that future editions of DSM will contain a better-defined category of obsessive-compulsive spectrum disorders.

Should Somatoform Disorders Be Moved to Different Sections of DSM?

According to DSM-IV-TR, "the common feature of the Somatoform Disorders is the presence of physical symptoms that suggest a general medical condition (hence, the term *somatoform*)" (American Psychiatric Association

2000, p. 485). The somatoform disorders section, which was new to DSM-III, consists of somatization disorder, undifferentiated somatoform disorder, conversion disorder, pain disorder, hypochondriasis, and BDD. Also according to DSM-IV-TR, grouping these disorders together in a single section "is based on clinical utility (i.e., the need to exclude occult general medical conditions or substance-induced etiologies for the bodily symptoms) rather than on assumptions regarding shared etiology or mechanism" (p. 485).

The somatoform disorders—although similar in content (i.e., a focus on the body)—seem quite dissimilar in form and are likely to have distinct etiologies. The "forms" or "structures" of BDD and at least one variant of hypochondriasis are characterized by prominent obsessions and compulsive behaviors, as well as other similarities to OCD (Fallon et al. 1991; Hollander and Phillips 1993; Phillips et al. 1998). Indeed, it is sometimes difficult to differentiate hypochondriasis from the somatic obsessions of OCD. Complicating this picture, however, is that some of the somatoform disorders appear heterogeneous; for example, another clinical variant of hypochondriasis appears more similar to somatization disorder or depressive disorders than to OCD (Barsky et al. 1986; Noyes et al. 1994, 1997; Tyrer et al. 1980).

The structure, or form, of conversion disorder is quite different from that of BDD and hypochondriasis. Rather than consisting of prominent obsessions and compulsions, conversion disorder consists of symptoms or deficits affecting voluntary motor or sensory function, such as paralysis, aphonia, or double vision. And in contrast to the marked distress often experienced by patients with BDD (Phillips 1991), patients with conversion disorder often have a lack of concern about their bodily symptoms (*la belle indifférence*). Although the mechanism by which conversion symptoms develop is not entirely clear, dissociation appears to play an important role (Martin 1992). Indeed, it has been argued that conversion disorder shares essential phenomenological features with the dissociative disorders and should be placed in that section of DSM (Kihlstrom 1992; McHugh and Slavney 1998; Nemiah 1991). In *The ICD-10 Classification of Mental and Behavioural Disorders* (World Health Organization 1992), conversion disorder and the dissociative disorders are placed together in a superordinate category termed *dissociative (conversion) disorders*. A similar approach was used in DSM-II, in which conversion and dissociative disorders were two subtypes of hysterical neurosis, a union "that had its roots in antiquity" (Martin 1996; Nemiah 1991). In DSM-III, these disorders were split into the somatoform and dissociative disorders. During the process of constructing DSM-IV, moving conversion disorder back to the dissociative disorders section was considered, reflecting evidence that conversion and dissociative symptoms often co-occur and may have a related pathogenesis (American Psychiatric Association 1991; Martin 1996). However, this change was not made, because it was argued that conversion disorder appears to be related to certain somatoform disorders, particularly somatization and pain disorder (Martin 1992), and that keeping conversion disorder in the somatoform section facilitates the differential diagnosis of somatic symptoms (Frances et al. 1995). This issue is far from resolved; some authors maintain that this decision was a mistake (Kihlstrom 1994).

The relationship between somatization disorder and other psychiatric disorders is even less clear. Comorbidity studies suggest a relationship with conversion disorder, dissociative disorders, depressive disorders, panic disorder, substance-related disorders, and cluster B personality disorders (Cloninger et al. 1986, 1997; Hudziak et al. 1996; Saxe et al. 1994; Simon and VonKorff 1991; Stern et al. 1993). Family studies suggest a relationship with substance-related disorders and antisocial personality disorder (Cloninger et al. 1975).

At this time, research that sheds light on this nosological dilemma is very limited. Although we think it would be ideal to eliminate this grouping of disorders, it is not yet clear where they should be placed. As we concluded about the obsessive-compulsive spectrum hypothesis, data on the pathogenesis of these disorders are needed to guide such a change. We anticipate that when data become available, they will support disbanding this remarkably heterogeneous group of disorders and reclassifying them in a way that more accurately reflects their relationships with other disorders. It is likely that research findings will support classifying BDD with OCD, consistent with historical conceptualizations of BDD (Phillips 1991). The OCD-like variant of hypochondriasis may be classified with the obsessive-compulsive spectrum disorders, whereas its somatization disorder–like variant may be classified with somatization disorder. We anticipate that conversion disorder will be classified with the dissociative disorders, reflecting their common historical roots and likely similar pathogenesis. The classification of somatization disorder is more complex; the most accurate placement may prove to be with the cluster B personality disorders.

Should Delusional and Nondelusional Variants of Disorders Be Combined?

Should delusional and nondelusional variants of disorders be classified as a single disorder, spanning a spectrum of insight, or should they be classified as distinct disorders? For example, does Ms. A's preoccupation with her nose, which was sometimes delusional and sometimes not, constitute a single disorder or two disorders? In DSM-IV, nondelusional BDD is classified as a somatoform disorder, whereas delusional BDD is classified as a psychotic disorder—a type of delusional disorder, somatic type. Delusional hypochondriasis is classified as delusional disorder, somatic type; and delusional OCD is classified as psychotic disorder not otherwise specified or delusional disorder, unspecified type.

Although these disorders' psychotic and nonpsychotic forms are classified separately, in some respects their classification is handled inconsistently (see Table 3–2). One inconsistency is DSM-IV-TR's statement that delusional OCD, unlike delusional BDD or hypochondriasis, may be classified as either delusional disorder or psychotic disorder not otherwise specified. Another inconsistency is that whereas BDD and OCD may be double coded with their delusional disorder variant (i.e., patients with delusional symptoms may receive both diagnoses), reflecting the possibility that their delusional and nondelusional forms constitute the same disorder, this is not noted as an option for hypochondriasis. (An additional problem is that it is unclear whether delusional and nondelusional BDD or OCD should be double coded; the *may* in the DSM-IV-TR text is ambiguous.) Still another inconsistency is that OCD and hypochondriasis have a "poor insight" specifier but BDD does not, even though BDD is more often characterized by poor insight than is OCD (Eisen et al. 1999). The criteria for hypochondriasis further differentiate delusional and nondelusional forms of the disorder with criterion C, which specifies that "the belief in criterion A is not of delusional intensity" (American Psychiatric Association 2000, p. 507); this is not done for the other disorders. DSM-IV-TR is silent on insight in anorexia nervosa, although most clinicians would recognize that insight is often poor and some patients are delusional.

As shown in Table 3–2, the mood disorders are handled quite differently. The psychotic variant of major depression or bipolar disorder is classified as a subtype of the mood disorder (e.g., major depression with psychotic features) rather than as a separate disorder in the psychotic disorders section (although questions were raised during the planning of DSM-IV about whether psychotic depression should be classified separately from nonpsychotic depression [Schatzberg and Rothschild 1996]). Should the major depression model be adopted for these other disorders?

Using BDD as an example, although its delusional and nondelusional variants are classified separately, earlier authors noted that BDD's precursor, dysmorphophobia, encompassed both nonpsychotic (or neurotic) and psychotic thinking (Phillips 1991). In keeping with this historical perspective, available data indicate that BDD and its delusional disorder variant do not significantly differ in terms of demographics, phenomenology, course, associated psychopathology, family history, or treatment response, although the delusional variant appears to be a more severe form of the dis-

TABLE 3–2. Classification of delusional and nondelusional forms of disorders in DSM-IV-TR

Disorder	Delusional and nondelusional forms classified together	Separate delusional disorder variant	Psychotic disorder NOS	Double coded	"Poor insight" specifier	Intensity specification
BDD		X		X		
OCD		X	X	X	X	
Hypochondriasis		X			X	X
Anorexia nervosa						
Psychotic mood disorder	X					

Note.   NOS=not otherwise specified; BDD=body dysmorphic disorder; OCD=obsessive-compulsive disorder.

order (Phillips et al. 1994). Of note, delusional BDD, like nondelusional BDD, appears to respond to serotonin reuptake inhibitors (Hollander et al. 1999; Phillips et al. 2001, 2002). This view implies that delusionality is a dimensional construct, with insight occurring on a continuum and sometimes changing over time (Phillips et al. 1994; Strauss 1969). Changes in insight may occur in response to treatment or be triggered by the social environment or stress (Phillips et al. 1998). It is highly unlikely that a given patient, such as Ms. A, would have one disorder at one moment and another disorder at another. The more parsimonious explanation is that she has a single disorder characterized by a spectrum of insight.

In the OCD literature as well, insight has been noted to vary on a continuum ranging from good insight to delusional thinking (Eisen and Rasmussen 1993; Insel and Akiskal 1986; Solyom et al. 1985). As in BDD, it can be difficult to distinguish between different levels of insight, and insight may vary and be situation dependent (Foa et al. 1996). A study that compared OCD patients with and without insight found that the two groups were generally similar in terms of demographic and clinical characteristics (Eisen and Rasmussen 1993). In addition, most studies suggest that patients with poor insight respond as well to behavior therapy as patients with good insight (Lelliott and Marks 1987; Lelliott et al. 1988; Salkovskis and Wernike 1985). Preliminary evidence suggests that the same is true for response to serotonin reuptake inhibitors (Eisen et al. 2001).

Progress in resolving this diagnostic dilemma has been limited by the lack of widely used, validated instruments to assess delusionality in psychiatric disorders other than schizophrenia, reflecting how a paucity of assessment tools can impede advances in classification. Research has also been compromised by the fact that delusions are multidimensional concepts (Kendler et al. 1983) and that the very definition of delusions is a subject of some controversy (M. Spitzer 1990). Further studies using reliable and valid scales to assess delusionality (see, for example, Eisen et al. 1998) are needed to clarify the relationship between delusional and nondelusional variants of disorders. Investigation of the pathogenesis of these disorders' psychotic and nonpsychotic forms is also needed, as is investigation into whether there is a continuum between normal beliefs and delusions.

We anticipate that future research will show that BDD, OCD, hypochondriasis, and anorexia nervosa are characterized by a spectrum of insight and that the subtype model—with and without psychotic features— used to classify mood disorders will prove more valid and clinically useful than the current schema. The model proposed (although not fully adopted) for OCD in DSM-IV—"with insight," "with overvalued ideas," and "with delusional thinking"—is even more appealing, because it allows for more gradations in insight. In our view, this change should be made consistently in DSM-V, assuming such consistency is supported by emerging empirical evidence. This would allow double coding to be deleted and the other classification inconsistencies shown in Table 3–2 to be eliminated.

Should DSM Include a Section of Stress-Related Disorders?

During the revision process leading up to DSM-IV, a debated option was to move PTSD from the anxiety disorders section into a newly created section of "stress-related disorders" (American Psychiatric Association 1991; Davidson et al. 1996). However, it was unclear which disorders should be members of this new category. One proposal included PTSD and acute stress disorder, whereas a second proposal also included adjustment disorder, similar to the category "reaction to severe stress and adjustment disorders" in *The ICD-10 Classification of Mental and Behavioural Disorders* (World Health Organization 1992). A third, broader proposal included all three of these disorders plus pathological grief and uncomplicated bereavement. Yet another proposal was to create a new category called *disorders of extreme stress not otherwise specified*, a residual category for responses following trauma that do not meet criteria for acute stress disorder or PTSD. (It was also proposed that PTSD be classified with the dissociative disorders [Davidson and Foa, 1991a, 1991b; Davidson et al. 1996].)

The DSM-IV work group's major rationale for proposing that a section of stress-related disorders be created was to emphasize stress as "a common etiologic factor" (American Psychiatric Association 1991). Indeed, a major advantage of this proposal is that it attempts to move DSM toward an etiologically based classification system. Other advantages cited by the work group (American Psychiatric Association 1991; Davidson et al. 1996) were that classifying stress-related disorders together would facilitate differential diagnosis and that grouping PTSD, acute stress disorder, and adjustment disorder (the second proposal in the previous paragraph) would make DSM more comparable to *The ICD-10 Classification of Mental and Behavioural Disorders* (World Health Organization 1992).

The major limitation of this proposal is that although stress clearly plays an important role in the onset of these disorders (Davidson and Foa 1991b), it is not their only cause. The etiology of PTSD, for example, is multifactorial. Factors such as neuroticism may influence whether exposure to a trauma results in PTSD (Breslau et al. 1991; McFarlane 1988). There are also significant genetic influences on symptom liability; one study found that even after adjusting for differences in combat exposure, genetic factors accounted for 13%–30% of the variance in liability for symptoms in the reexperiencing cluster, 30%–34% for symptoms in the avoidance cluster, and 28%–32% for symptoms in the arousal cluster (Lyons et al. 1993; True et al. 1993). An etiologically based classification would need to account for genetic, temperamental, and other etiological factors in addition to stress.

Another drawback to this proposal is that although some research suggests a special etiological connection between a traumatic event and PTSD (Davidson and Foa 1991a), stress is nonetheless nonspecific as a risk factor for psychiatric illness, playing an etiological role in many disorders, not just the proposed members of a stress-related category. One study involving depressed women, for example, found that a history of recent stressful life events was a powerful predictor of an episode of major depression in the preceding year, accounting for 39% of the variance in the liability for a depressive episode (Kendler et al. 1993). This study determined that more distant stressors also contributed to a depressive episode, a finding that raises the complex question of whether a category of stress-related disorders would be based on more recent stressors, more distant stressors, or both. Approximately 50% of psychiatric inpatients report a childhood history of severe chronic physical and/or sexual abuse (Beck and van der Kolk 1987; Bryer et al. 1987), which suggests a lack of specificity between reported childhood trauma and psychiatric disorders (van der Kolk and van der Hart 1989). This view of stress as one of several etiological variables is reflected in the "vulnerability–stress" model of psychiatric illnesses such as schizophrenia (Norman and Malla 1993).

Although the DSM-IV work group recommended that PTSD, acute stress response, and disorders of extreme stress not otherwise specified be placed in a separate category of stress- or trauma-related disorders (Davidson et al. 1996), this change was not made, because research on the relationship among these disorders did not appear sufficiently advanced to justify reclassification (Davidson and Foa 1991b). It seems premature to regroup these disorders to reflect the etiological role of stress, given that stress is not the only etiological factor and is nonspecific as a risk factor. However, it is likely that future research, including advances in the neurosciences and in the understanding of environmental risk factors, may eventually justify such an approach.

Research Needed to Solve Organizational Dilemmas

To solve the organizational diagnostic dilemmas discussed in this chapter, and to create a more rational basis for organizing DSM as a whole, the following research is needed:

1. *Clarification and refinement of phenotypes.* Phenomenological similarities and differences are an indispensable starting point for determining the relationship among disorders (Kendell 1984). Accurate phenomenological description increases the likelihood that etiology will be elucidated (Kendell 1989). Some of the putative obsessive-compulsive spectrum disorders and the delusional versus nondelusional forms of disorders, for example, have undergone surprisingly little investigation, even at the phenomenological level.

2. *Research on other domains.* A convergence of data from multiple domains (e.g., family history, course of illness, and treatment response) is also needed (Kendell 1989). The criteria of Robins and Guze (1990) remain relevant today.

3. *Neurobiological studies.* To organize DSM optimally, data on etiology and pathophysiology—in particular, neurobiological data (such as imaging findings, genetic data, and neurochemical findings)—are critical. Symptoms do not necessarily correspond to etiology, and phenotypic homogeneity does not guarantee biological homogeneity. Neurobiological data will help validate the boundaries of diagnostic entities and subtypes, establish groupings of etiologically related disorders, and split groups of disorders established on the basis of phenomenology.

   An important irony is that valid data on pathogenesis can be obtained only by using accurate, valid, and adequately homogeneous clinical phenotypes (see item 1). This important point was noted as long ago as 1942: "The part played by heredity in the development of the psychoneuroses is one of the fundamental unsolved problems in psychiatry.... But the chief difficulty is to define the condition the heredity of which one is attempting to trace" (Brown 1942). More recently, Smoller and Tsuang (1998) made a similar point: "With recent advances in molecular genetics, the rate-limiting step in identifying susceptibility genes for psychiatric disorders has become phenotype definition" (p. 1152). If diagnostic entities are not etiologically homogeneous, searching for modes of transmission is similar to the genetic study of dropsy (Knowles et al. 1999). Phenomenology and knowledge of neurobiology and genetics are linked through an important iterative process, with refinement of the phenotype critically important for genetic studies.

4. *Research on dimensional approaches to classification.* The dimensional approach to classification is potentially powerful, and it is possible that the future classification system will include dimensions in addition to or instead of categories. For example, a study of the phenotypic and genetic structure of personality disorder traits supported a dimensional classification of personality disorder shaped by multiple distinct genetic factors (Livesley et al. 1998). Future studies relevant to classification,

including genetic studies, should incorporate dimensional measures (Greenberg et al. 1998; Moldin et al. 1991; Pauls 1993; Smoller and Tsuang 1998).

Radical Reorganization: Potential Challenges and Pitfalls

A challenge that will be based on judgment more than data is what amount of data on pathogenesis will be needed before DSM is reorganized. What are the criteria that will be used? Criteria are needed to establish how similar two disorders (e.g., hypochondriasis and OCD) or two forms of disorders (e.g., delusional and nondelusional OCD) should be before deeming them the same or related disorders. How many imaging or genetics studies—and how many replication studies—will be needed to reorganize DSM? How much information on environmental determinants of disorders will be needed? Whether and how to incorporate these types of data into DSM will be the greatest challenge faced by future DSM task forces.

Another challenge is posed by the fact that psychiatric disorders do not have clear-cut inheritance patterns (Knowles et al. 1999); they are likely complex disorders, involving multiple susceptibility genes of small effect combined with multiple environmental risk factors (Barondes 1999; Greenberg et al. 1998; McInnis 1997; Plomin 1990; Reiss et al. 1991). The single-gene autosomal dominant transmission demonstrated for Huntington's disease is unlikely to be replicated for many psychiatric disorders, if any. Alzheimer's disease illustrates this complexity. A number of specific genes have been identified as critical in the development of many cases of Alzheimer's disease, with mutations in different genes appearing to cause similar clinical and pathological Alzheimer's phenotypes (Knowles et al. 1999; Lendon et al. 1997; Plassman and Breitner 1997). Furthermore, the influence of Alzheimer's disease genes may be modified in the presence of other relevant genes (Plassman and Breitner 1997), as well as environmental influences, which may accelerate or delay onset of dementia symptoms associated with specific predisposing genes, or reduce expression of such symptoms (Breitner and Welsh 1995; Mayeux et al. 1995; Plassman and Breitner 1997). How would this complexity be reflected in a diagnostic manual that must be clinically useful?

Another challenge is the question of whether a person with the genotype for an illness should receive the diagnosis if the phenotype is not expressed—for example, because of incomplete penetrance (Lander and Schrok 1994; Tsuang et al. 1993). In the case of Alzheimer's disease, neuropathological changes may occur decades before symptoms are apparent clinically (Plassman and Breitner 1997). Phenotypic and genetic heterogeneity are complicating factors in other disorders as well (Mullan and Murray 1989; O'Donovan and McGuffin 1991; Tsuang et al. 1993), just as they are in medical illnesses (Fananapazir 1999).

Given these complexities, it may be difficult to organize future DSMs on the basis of etiology. DSM may retain a syndrome-based classification system that is informed by knowledge of pathogenesis—a system with, for example, etiologically or pathophysiologically based subtypes, as is currently the case with Alzheimer's disease. Ultimately, because DSM is a manual for clinicians, it must have clinical utility.

DSM-V: An Awkward Transition

It would be premature to rearrange DSM now on the basis of etiology and pathophysiology; however, this will likely be possible in the future. Ultimately, as these data become available, they should influence how individual disorders are defined and how DSM is organized. The question for the next few editions of DSM is whether there will be enough data to make radical changes. These manuals will take shape during the decades when knowledge of pathogenesis will take a quantum leap forward. The change from a syndrome-based classification system to one based on pathogenesis—if such a change occurs—will be gradual, because neurobiological research will progress at different rates for different disorders. There will likely be an awkward transition phase in which some, but not other, disorders may be reclassified according to pathogenesis. It has been said that "there is never a good time to introduce a new diagnostic system; it is always both too soon and too late" (Frances et al. 1991, p. 411). We anticipate that the next few editions of DSM will be introduced at a particularly awkward time.

Potential Solutions

There are several conservative ways to incorporate data on pathogenesis as they become available. Neurobiological data could be included in the laboratory section of the text (as is currently done for narcolepsy) or under the heading "Predisposing Factors," also in the text. This approach would allow new knowledge to be integrated into future DSMs but would not advance the classification system. Another approach would be to expand Axis III to include neurobiological data (e.g., genetic or neuroimaging data), or to create a separate axis for such data. This approach would facilitate integration of this information into clinicians' thinking about patients but also would not advance the classification system. A more radical solution would be to integrate neurobiological data, as they become available, into diagnostic criteria and the organization of disorders.

As noted in "Radical Reorganization," a problem with the more radical solutions is that it is unclear when such changes should be made. How much information is enough? One solution to this problem, which we favor and which was considered during the planning of DSM-IV, is to have a separate DSM-like manual for researchers. This approach would be similar to that of *The ICD-10 Classification of Mental and Behavioural Disorders* (World Health Organization 1992), in which research diagnostic criteria are provided in a different manual than the manual of official clinical criteria. This DSM-like manual could include proposed diagnostic criteria, axes, subtypes, or new groupings of disorders based on recent findings on pathogenesis, such as genetic data, neuroimaging findings, or biological markers (e.g., eye-tracking abnormalities in schizophrenia or lactate sensitivity in panic disorder). In making use of emerging information on etiopathology for this purpose, standards of evidence should be relatively rigorous. Consistency, specificity, and coherence with results of other approaches are hallmarks of valid associations, as Hill (1965) pointed out in his classic article on case-control studies in medicine. This manual could also include operational definitions of psychopathological dimensions (e.g., "anxiety diathesis") in addition to categorical concepts. This proposed manual would be biologically informed and sensitive to environmental risk factors. It would be a work in progress that would have the advantage of reflecting recent research advances without prematurely changing the official diagnostic criteria, as well as the advantage of stimulating research that would ultimately inform the clinical manual. One potential criticism of this approach, however, is that it would widen the gap between research and clinical practice, although efforts could be made to enhance the consistency between these classification systems. Another potential problem is that this approach could be viewed as official sanctioning of specific research agendas.

An additional recommendation is to avoid combining disorders prematurely, without strong supporting scientific evidence. Until more is known about disorders' pathogenesis, it is better to split (i.e., describe a larger number of categories) than combine, so that the putative disorders are studied and important differences between them are not missed. Studies involving homogeneous populations have greater statistical power than those involving heterogeneous populations. The history of psychiatric classification is replete with examples of diagnostic and treatment errors attributable to premature lumping (e.g., combining schizophrenia and manic-depressive illness). We are not advocating the addition of more disorders so much as cautioning that lumping should not be done prematurely. Once there is a better understanding of these disorders' pathogenesis, they can be combined in an informed and valid way.

In conclusion, the current diagnostic groupings are a useful heuristic but should not be considered a definitive reflection of the relationships among disorders. These groupings are temporary and are likely to change radically in upcoming decades as pathogenesis becomes known. Ideally, the DSM edifice of the future will be founded in pathogenesis, with the organization of disorders reflecting the etiological and pathophysiological relationships among them.

References

American Psychiatric Association: Diagnostic and Statistical Manual: Mental Disorders. Washington, DC, American Psychiatric Association, 1952

American Psychiatric Association: Diagnostic and Statistical Manual of Mental Disorders, 2nd Edition. Washington, DC, American Psychiatric Association, 1968

American Psychiatric Association: Diagnostic and Statistical Manual of Mental Disorders, 3rd Edition. Washington, DC, American Psychiatric Association, 1980

American Psychiatric Association: Diagnostic and Statistical Manual of Mental Disorders, 3rd Edition, Revised. Washington, DC, American Psychiatric Association, 1987

American Psychiatric Association: DSM-IV Options Book: Work in Progress. Washington, DC, American Psychiatric Association, 1991

American Psychiatric Association: Diagnostic and Statistical Manual of Mental Disorders, 4th Edition. Washington, DC, American Psychiatric Association, 1994

American Psychiatric Association: Diagnostic and Statistical Manual of Mental Disorders, 4th Edition, Revised. Washington, DC, American Psychiatric Association, 2000

Barondes SH: An agenda for psychiatric genetics. Arch Gen Psychiatry 56:549–552, 1999

Barsky AJ, Wyshak G, Klerman GL: Hypochondriasis: an evaluation of the DSM-III criteria in medical outpatients. Arch Gen Psychiatry 43:493–500, 1986

Beck JC, van der Kolk B: Reports of childhood incest and current behavior of chronically hospitalized psychotic women. Am J Psychiatry 144:1474–1476, 1987

Bienvenu OJ, Samuels JF, Riddle MA, et al: The relationship of obsessive-compulsive disorder to possible spectrum disorders: results from a family study. Biol Psychiatry 48:287–293, 2000

Breitner JCS, Welsh KA: Genes and recent developments in the epidemiology of Alzheimer's disease and related dementia. Epidemiol Rev 17:39–47, 1995

Breslau N, Davis GC, Andreski P, et al: Traumatic events and posttraumatic stress disorder in an urban population of young adults. Arch Gen Psychiatry 48:216–222, 1991

Brown F: Heredity in the psychoneuroses. Proc R Soc Med 35:785–790, 1942

Bryer JB, Nelson BA, Miller JB, et al: Childhood sexual and physical abuse as factors in adult psychiatric illness. Am J Psychiatry 144:1426–1430, 1987

Clark LA, Watson D, Reynolds S: Diagnosis and classification of psychopathology: challenges to the current system and future directions. Annu Rev Psychol 46:121–153, 1995

Cloninger CR, Reich T, Guze SB: The multifactorial model of disease transmission, III: familial relationships between sociopathy and hysteria (Briquet's syndrome). Br J Psychiatry 1127:23–32, 1975

Cloninger CR, Martin RL, Guze SB, et al: A prospective follow-up and family study of somatization in men and women. Am J Psychiatry 143:873–878, 1986

Cloninger CR, Bayon C, Przybeck TR: Epidemiology and Axis I comorbidity of antisocial personality, in Handbook of Antisocial Behavior. Edited by Stoff DM, Maser JD, Breiling J. New York, Wiley, 1997, pp 12–21

Compton WM, Guze SB: The neo-Kraepelinian revolution in psychiatric diagnosis. Eur Arch Psychiatry Clin Neurosci 245:196–201, 1995

Davidson JRT, Foa EB: Diagnostic issues in posttraumatic stress disorder: considerations for the DSM-IV. J Abnorm Psychol 100:346–355, 1991a

Davidson JRT, Foa EB: Refining criteria for posttraumatic stress disorder. Hosp Community Psychiatry 42:259–261, 1991b

Davidson JRT, Foa EB, Blank AS, et al: Posttraumatic stress disorder, in DSM-IV Sourcebook, Vol 2. Edited by Widiger TA, Frances AJ, Pincus HA, et al. Washington, DC, American Psychiatric Association, 1996, pp 577–605

Eisen JL, Rasmussen SA: Obsessive compulsive disorder with psychotic features. J Clin Psychiatry 54:373–379, 1993

Eisen JL, Phillips KA, Baer L, et al: The Brown Assessment of Beliefs Scale: reliability and validity. Am J Psychiatry 155:102–108, 1998

Eisen JL, Phillips KA, Rasmussen SA: Obsessions and delusions: the relationship between obsessive compulsive disorder and the psychotic disorders. Psychiatric Annals 29:515–522, 1999

Eisen JL, Rasmussen SA, Phillips KA, et al: Insight and treatment outcome in obsessive-compulsive disorder. Compr Psychiatry 42:494–497, 2001

Fallon BA, Javitch JA, Hollander E, et al: Hypochondriasis and obsessive compulsive disorder: overlaps in diagnosis and treatment. J Clin Psychiatry 52:457–460, 1991

Fananapazir L: Advances in molecular genetics and management of hypertrophic cardiomyopathy. JAMA 281:1746–1752, 1999

Faraone SV, Kremen WS, Lyons MJ, et al: Diagnostic accuracy and linkage analysis: how useful are schizophrenia spectrum phenotypes? Am J Psychiatry 152:1286–1290, 1995

Foa WV, Jenike M, Kozak M, et al: Obsessive-compulsive disorder, in DSM-IV Sourcebook, Vol 2. Edited by Widiger TA, Frances AJ, Pincus HA, et al. Washington, DC, American Psychiatric Association, 1996, pp 549–575

Frances A[J], Pincus HA, Widiger TA, et al: DSM-IV: work in progress. Am J Psychiatry 147:1439–1448, 1990

Frances AJ, First MB, Widiger TA, et al: An A to Z guide to DSM-IV conundrums. J Abnorm Psychol 100:407–412, 1991

Frances A[J], Mack AH, Ross R, et al: The DSM-IV classification and psychopharmacology, in Psychopharmacology: The Fourth Generation of Progress. Edited by Bloom FE, Kupfer DJ. New York, Raven, 1995, pp 823–828

Greenberg BD, McMahon FJ, Murphy DL: Serotonin transporter candidate gene studies in affective disorders and personality: promises and potential pitfalls. Mol Psychiatry 3:186–189, 1998

Hill AB: The environment and disease: association or causation? Proc R Soc Med 58:295–300, 1965

Hollander E: Introduction, in Obsessive-Compulsive-Related Disorders. Edited by Hollander E. Washington, DC, American Psychiatric Press, 1993, pp 1–16

Hollander E, Allen A, Kwon J, et al: Clomipramine vs desipramine crossover trial in body dysmorphic disorder: selective efficacy of a serotonin reuptake inhibitor in imagined ugliness. Arch Gen Psychiatry 56:1033–1039, 1999

Hudson JI, Pope HG Jr: Affective spectrum disorder: does antidepressant response identify a family of disorders with a common pathophysiology? Am J Psychiatry 147:553–564, 1990

Hudziak JJ, Boffeli TJ, Kriesman JJ, et al: Clinical study of the relation of borderline personality disorder to Briquet's syndrome (hysteria), somatization disorder, antisocial personality disorder, and substance abuse disorders. Am J Psychiatry 153:1598–1606, 1996

Insel TR, Akiskal H: Obsessive-compulsive disorder with psychotic features: a phenomenologic analysis. Am J Psychiatry 12:1527–1533, 1986

Kendell RE: Reflections on psychiatric classification—for the architects of DSM-IV and ICD-10. Integr Psychiatry March–April:43–47, 1984

Kendell RE: Clinical validity, in The Validity of Psychiatric Diagnosis. Edited by Robins LN, Barrett JE. New York, Raven, 1989, pp 305–323

Kendell RE: Relationship between the DSM-IV and the ICD-10. J Abnorm Psychol 100:297–301, 1991

Kendler KS, Glazer WM, Morgenstern H: Dimensions of delusional experience. Am J Psychiatry 140:466–469, 1983

Kendler KS, Kessler RC, Neale MC, et al: The prediction of major depression in women: toward an integrated etiologic model. Am J Psychiatry 150:1139–1148, 1993

Kendler KS, Walters EE, Neale MC, et al: The structure of the genetic and environmental risk factors for six major psychiatric disorders in women. Arch Gen Psychiatry 52:374–383, 1995

Kihlstrom JF: Dissociative and conversion disorders, in Cognitive Science and Clinical Disorders. Edited by Stein DJ, Young JE. San Diego, CA, Academic Press, 1992, pp 247–270

Kihlstrom JF: One hundred years of hysteria, in Dissociation. Edited by Lynn SJ, Rhue JW. New York, Guilford, 1994, pp 365–394

Klein DF: Foreword, in Obsessive-Compulsive-Related Disorders. Edited by Hollander E. Washington, DC, American Psychiatric Press, 1993, pp xi–xvii

Knowles JA, Kaufmann CA, Rieder RO: Genetics, in The American Psychiatric Press Textbook of Psychiatry, 3rd Edition. Edited by Hales RE, Yudofsky SC, Talbott JA. Washington, DC, American Psychiatric Press, 1999, pp 35–82

Lander ES, Schrok NJ: Genetic dissection of complex traits. Science 265:2037–2048, 1994

Leckman JF, Walker DE, Goodman WK, et al: "Just right" perceptions associated with compulsive behavior in Tourette's syndrome. Am J Psychiatry 151:675–680, 1994

Lelliott PT, Marks I: Management of obsessive compulsive rituals associated with delusions, hallucinations, and depression: a case report. Behavioral Psychotherapy 15:77–87, 1987

Lelliott PT, Noshirvani HF, Basoglu M, et al: Obsessive-compulsive beliefs and treatment outcome. Psychol Med 18:697–702, 1988

Lendon CL, Ashall F, Goate AM: Exploring the etiology of Alzheimer disease using molecular genetics. JAMA 277:825–831, 1997

Livesley WJ, Jang KL, Vernon PA: Phenotypic and genetic structure of traits delineating personality disorder. Arch Gen Psychiatry 55:941–948, 1998

Lyons MJ, Goldberg J, Eisen SA, et al: Do genes influence exposure to trauma? a twin study of combat. Am J Med Genet 48:22–27, 1993

Mack AH, Forman L, Brown R, et al: A brief history of psychiatric classification. Psychiatr Clin North Am 17:515–523, 1994

Marazziti D, Dell'Osso L, Presta S, et al: Platelet [3H]paroxetine binding in patients with OCD-related disorders. Psychiatry Res 89:223–228, 1999

Martin RL: Diagnostic issues for conversion disorder. Hosp Community Psychiatry 43:771–773, 1992

Martin RL: Conversion disorder, proposed autonomic arousal disorder, and pseudocyesis, in DSM-IV Sourcebook, Vol 2. Edited by Widiger TA, Frances AJ, Pincus HA, et al. Washington, DC, American Psychiatric Association, 1996, pp 893–914

Mayeux R, Ottman R, Maestre G, et al: Synergistic effects of traumatic head injury and apolipoprotein-epsilon 4 in patients with Alzheimer's disease. Neurology 45:555–557, 1995

McElroy SL, Phillips KA, Keck PE Jr: Obsessive-compulsive spectrum disorder. J Clin Psychiatry 55 (suppl):33–51, 1994

McFarlane AC: The longitudinal course of posttraumatic morbidity: the range of outcomes and their predictors. J Nerv Ment Dis 176:30–39, 1988

McHugh PR, Slavney PR: The Perspective of Psychiatry, 2nd Edition. Baltimore, MD, Johns Hopkins University Press, 1998

McInnis MG: Recent advances in the genetics of bipolar disorder. Psychiatric Annals 27:482–488, 1997

Moldin SO, Gottesman II, Rice JP, et al: Replicated psychometric correlates of schizophrenia. Am J Psychiatry 148:762–767, 1991

Morey LC: Classification of mental disorder as a collection of hypothetical constructs. J Abnorm Psychol 100:289–293, 1991

Mullan MJ, Murray RM: The impact of molecular genetics on our understanding of the psychoses. Br J Psychiatry 154:591–595, 1989

Nemiah JC: Dissociation, conversion, and somatization, in Review of Psychiatry, Vol 10. Edited by Tasman A, Goldfinger SM. Washington, DC, American Psychiatric Press, 1991, pp 248–260

Norman RMG, Malla AK: Stressful life events and schizophrenia, I: a review of the research. Br J Psychiatry 162:161–166, 1993

Noyes R Jr, Kathol RG, Fisher MM, et al: Psychiatric comorbidity among patients with hypochondriasis. Gen Hosp Psychiatry 16:78–87, 1994

Noyes R Jr, Holt CS, Happel RL, et al: A family study of hypochondriasis. J Nerv Ment Dis 185:223–232, 1997

O'Donovan M, McGuffin P: Linkage and association studies, in Genetic Issues in Psychosocial Epidemiology. Edited by Tsuang MT, Kendler KS, Lyons MJ. New Brunswick, NJ, Rutgers University Press, 1991

Pauls DL: Behavioural disorders: lessons in linkage. Nat Genet 3:4–5, 1993

Pearlstein TB, Stone AB, Lund SA, et al: Comparison of fluoxetine, bupropion, and placebo in the treatment of premenstrual dysphoric disorder. J Clin Psychopharmacol 17:261–266, 1997

Phillips KA: Body dysmorphic disorder: the distress of imagined ugliness. Am J Psychiatry 148:1138–1149, 1991

Phillips KA, Hollander E: Body dysmorphic disorder, in DSM-IV Sourcebook, Vol 2. Edited by Widiger TA, Frances AJ, Pincus HA, et al. Washington, DC, American Psychiatric Association, 1996, pp 949–960

Phillips KA, McElroy SL, Keck PE Jr, et al: A comparison of delusional and non-delusional body dysmorphic disorder in 100 cases. Psychopharmacol Bull 30:179–186, 1994

Phillips KA, McElroy SL, Hudson JI, et al: Body dysmorphic disorder: an obsessive-compulsive spectrum disorder, a form of affective spectrum disorder, or both? J Clin Psychiatry 56 (suppl 4):41–51, 1995

Phillips KA, Gunderson CG, Mallya G, et al: A comparison study of body dysmorphic disorder and obsessive-compulsive disorder. J Clin Psychiatry 59:568–575, 1998

Phillips KA, McElroy SL, Dwight MM, et al: Delusionality and response to open-label fluvoxamine in body dysmorphic disorder. J Clin Psychiatry 62:87–91, 2001

Phillips KA, Albertini RS, Rasmussen SA: A randomized placebo-controlled trial of fluoxetine in body dysmorphic disorder. Arch Gen Psychiatry 59:381–388, 2002

Plassman BL, Breitner JCS: The genetics of dementia in late life. Psychiatr Clin North Am 20:59–76, 1997

Plomin R: The role of inheritance in behavior. Science 248:183–188, 1990

Preskorn SH: Beyond DSM-IV: what is the cart and what is the horse? Psychiatric Annals 25:53–62, 1995

Price LH, Goddard AW, Barr LC, et al: Pharmacological challenges in anxiety disorders, in Psychopharmacology: The Fourth Generation of Progress. Edited by Bloom FE, Kupfer DJ. New York, Raven, 1995, pp 1311–1324

Rasmussen SA: Obsessive compulsive spectrum disorders. J Clin Psychiatry 55:89–91, 1994

Rauch SL: Advances in neuroimaging: how might they influence our diagnostic classification scheme? Harv Rev Psychiatry 4:159–162, 1996

Rauch SL, Baxter LR Jr: Neuroimaging in obsessive-compulsive disorder and related disorders, in Obsessive Compulsive Disorders: Practical Management, 3rd Edition. Edited by Jenike MJ, Baer L, Minichiello WE. St. Louis, MO, Mosby, 1998, pp 289–317

Rauch SL, Savage CR: Investigating cortico-striatal pathophysiology in obsessive-compulsive disorders: procedural learning and imaging probes, in Obsessive-Compulsive Disorder: Contemporary Issues in Treatment. Edited by Goodman WK, Rudorfer MV, Maser JD. Mahwah, NJ, Erlbaum, 2000, pp 133–156

Reiss D, Plomin R, Hetherington EM: Genetics and psychiatry: an unheralded window on the environment. Am J Psychiatry 148:283–290, 1991

Richter MA, Summerfeldt LJ, Joffe RT, et al: The Tridimensional Personality Questionnaire in obsessive-compulsive disorder. Psychiatry Res 20:185–188, 1996

Robins E, Guze SB: Establishment of diagnostic validity in psychiatric illness: its application to schizophrenia. Am J Psychiatry 126:983–987, 1970

Salkovskis PM, Wernike HMC: Cognitive therapy of obsessive-compulsive disorder: treating treatment failures. Behavioral Psychotherapy 13:243–255, 1985

Saxe GN, Chinman G, Berkowitz R, et al: Somatization in patients with dissociative disorders. Am J Psychiatry 151:1329–1334, 1994

Schatzberg AF, Rothschild AJ: Psychotic (delusional) major depression: should it be included as a distinct syndrome in DSM-IV? in DSM-IV Sourcebook, Vol 2. Edited by Widiger TA, Frances AJ, Pincus HA, et al. Washington, DC, American Psychiatric Association, 1996, pp 127–180

Simon GE, VonKorff M: Somatization and psychiatric disorder in the NIMH Epidemiologic Catchment Area study. Am J Psychiatry 148:1494–1500, 1991

Smoller JW, Tsuang MT: Panic and phobic anxiety: defining phenotypes for genetic studies. Am J Psychiatry 155:1152–1162, 1998

Solyom L, DiNicola VF, Phil M, et al: Is there an obsessive psychosis? aetiological and prognostic factors of an atypical form of obsessive-compulsive neurosis. Can J Psychiatry 30:372–380, 1985

Spitzer M: On defining delusions. Compr Psychiatry 31:377–397, 1990

Spitzer RS, Williams JBW: Classification of mental disorders and DSM-III, in Comprehensive Textbook of Psychiatry, 3rd Edition. Baltimore, MD, Williams & Wilkins, 1980, pp 1035–1072

Stein DJ: Neurobiology of the obsessive-compulsive spectrum disorders. Biol Psychiatry 47:296–304, 2000

Stern J, Murphy M, Bass C: Personality disorders in patients with somatization disorder: a controlled study. Br J Psychiatry 163:785–789, 1993

Strauss JS: Hallucinations and delusions as points on continua function: rating scale evidence. Arch Gen Psychiatry 21:581–586, 1969

Sullivan PF, Kendler KS: Typology of common psychiatric syndromes: an empirical study. Br J Psychiatry 173:312–319, 1998

Swedo SE, Leonard HL, Mittleman BB, et al: Identification of children with pediatric autoimmune neuropsychiatric disorders associated with streptococcal infections by a marker associated with rheumatic fever. Am J Psychiatry 154:110–112, 1997

Todd RD, Reich T: Linkage markers and validation of psychiatric nosology: toward an etiologic classification of psychiatric disorders, in The Validity of Psychiatric Diagnosis. Edited by Robins LN, Barrett JE. New York, Raven, 1989

True WR, Rice J, Eisen SA, et al: A twin study of genetic and environmental contributions to liability for posttraumatic stress symptoms. Arch Gen Psychiatry 50:257–264, 1993

Tsuang MT, Faraone SV, Lyons MJ: Identification of the phenotype in psychiatric genetics. Eur Arch Psychiatry Clin Neurosci 243:131–142, 1993

Tyrer P, Lee I, Alexander J: Awareness of cardiac function in anxious, phobic, and hypochondriacal patients. Psychol Med 10:171–174, 1980

van der Kolk BA, van der Hart O: Pierre Janet and the breakdown of adaptation in psychological trauma. Am J Psychiatry 146:1530–1540, 1989

World Health Organization: The ICD-10 Classification of Mental and Behavioural Disorders: Clinical Descriptions and Diagnostic Guidelines. Geneva, World Health Organization, 1992

CHAPTER 4

Laboratory Testing and Neuroimaging

Implications for Psychiatric Diagnosis and Practice

David C. Steffens, M.D., M.H.S.,
K. Ranga Rama Krishnan, M.B., Ch.B.

Laboratory tests or neuroimaging studies are commonly ordered as part of a psychiatric evaluation. Recognition of such testing in psychiatric practice necessitates consideration of its inclusion in the evolving diagnostic classification system. Currently, the only ancillary diagnostic tests referred to in DSM-IV-TR (American Psychiatric Association 2000) criteria sets are IQ tests for mental retardation and academic skills tests (e.g., tests of reading achievement) for specific learning disorders. Advances in the understanding of pathophysiology, genetics, and brain changes associated with a variety of psychiatric disorders have expanded diagnostic testing capabilities. Now that a number of laboratory and imaging tests are available, the time has come for consideration of testing in formal diagnostic schemes.

With the integration of laboratory tests and neuroimaging procedures into psychiatric practice, psychiatrists have begun to see some of the well-known difficulties associated with such testing in other medical specialties. Laboratory and imaging tests are best considered an extension of the process of clinical diagnosis. As such, they can provide valuable information for the treatment of patients. When used out of context, however, tests not only provide little information but also might hinder the diagnostic and

The writing of this chapter was supported in part by National Institute of Mental Health grants P50 MH60451 and R01 MH54846.

treatment process and increase the cost of management unnecessarily.

Laboratory and imaging tests are used in medicine for several reasons. Some tests are used for making diagnoses, others for predicting and monitoring treatment, and still others for determining prognosis. Tests employed for diagnosis are used in several ways—namely, to confirm a diagnosis, exclude a diagnosis, or screen patients (Ransahoff and Feinstein 1978).

There are two types of diagnostic tests: pathognomonic tests (i.e., tests that uniquely indicate a particular disease) and surrogate tests (i.e., tests that are potentially useful for differentiating or identifying a condition but are not used only for that particular condition) (Feinstein 1977). Tests for mutations in the presenilin 1 and presenilin 2 genes are examples of pathognomonic tests used to diagnose Alzheimer's disease (AD) in patients with early-onset dementia (Cruts et al. 1996). Surrogate tests, on the other hand, do not identify the disease. They identify something else, which one hopes will help identify the disease. Most of the difficulties associated with tests occur with the use of surrogate tests.

One such surrogate test is the dexamethasone suppression test (DST). After the introduction of the DST as a potentially useful diagnostic test for melancholia, the test began to be widely used, often indiscriminately. As with many new tests, the initial enthusiasm waned as the DST was used for varied disorders and in different settings. Soon questions arose about the utility of the DST as a diagnostic aid. For example, heterogeneity of clinical depression decreased the association between a diagnosis of depression and dexamethasone nonsuppression, making the test appear less sensitive for detecting depression. In addition, other factors such as concomitant dementia and withdrawal states were shown to produce positive DST results. Most of the difficulties commonly associated with surrogate tests also occur with the use of the DST (for a detailed discussion, see Krishnan et al. 1987).

In this chapter, we examine the general principles involved in ordering and interpreting diagnostic tests. We then focus on one particular illness, AD, and present the issues associated with diagnostic testing for that disease. We conclude with a discussion of the relationship between diagnostic testing and the psychiatric nomenclature and make some recommendations for DSM-V.

General Principles of Diagnostic Testing

A test can be evaluated at four levels (Galen 1982):

1. *Analytical level.* The technical aspects of a test (e.g., the precision, accuracy, detection sensitivity, and chemical specificity of the laboratory assay procedure) are considered at this level.

2. *Diagnostic performance level.* The focus at this level is on aspects such as the sensitivity, specificity, predictive value, and odds ratio of a test with respect to a particular diagnosis.
3. *Operational level.* At this level, the performance of a test is analyzed with reference to the clinical situation.
4. *Medical decision–making level.* The costs and benefits of a test are studied at this most important level.

Analytical Level

At the analytical level, the technical aspects, which include accuracy and precision, of a test are considered.

Accuracy refers to the tendency of test measurements to center around the true value. Using the DST as an example, let us consider the true plasma cortisol value of a sample to be 5 μg/dL. Suppose three methods are used to measure this sample, and six measurements are made using each method. If method 1 yields values of 5.1, 5.2, 5.1, 4.7, 5.0, and 4.9 μg/dL, method 2 yields values of 4.1, 4.2, 4.0, 4.1, 4.3, and 3.9 μg/dL, and method 3 yields values of 6.1, 6.2, 6.0, 5.9, 6.1, and 6.2 μg/dL, method 1 would be considered more accurate than the other two methods. The systematic error seen in the second and third assays is a test's bias. In statistical terms, a test's accuracy is measured by the proximity of the mean value to the true value.

Precision refers to the tendency of repeated measurements to yield the same results. For example, suppose the true plasma cortisol concentration of a sample is 5 μg/dL, and two methods are used to estimate the sample. If six measurements using method 1 yield results of 5.1, 5.2, 5.0, 4.9, 4.8, and 5.0 μg/dL, and method 2 yields results of 4.7, 4.3, 4.5, 5.0, 5.3, 5.5, and 5.7 μg/dL, method 1 is said to be more precise than method 2, even though the mean result with each method is 5 μg/dL. The precision of an assay often varies across the range of measured values. Usually, the optimal range of a reliable assay for hormones such as cortisol has a coefficient of variation of about 10%. Depending on the particular disease state being measured, the assay should be set up so that the highest level of precision is obtained for the range in which most of the results are likely to be seen and where maximum discrimination is needed.

Diagnostic Performance Level

At the diagnostic performance level, the technical aspects of testing populations for a particular diagnosis are studied. Examined at this level is how well a test performs with regard to a given sample of subjects. The test in question is compared with a *gold standard*, which describes the true state of the subject. In psychiatry, the gold standard is often a clinical examination that establishes the presence or absence of a particular diagnosis. The results of a study of a laboratory test's diagnostic performance are shown in Table 4–1. For the sake of simplicity, let us assume that the test is binary (i.e., has two possible outcomes [e.g., disease present or disease absent]).

As can be seen in Table 4–1, various definitions can be established on the basis of whether the disease is present or absent (according to the gold standard test) and whether the laboratory test results are positive or negative. If the laboratory test result is positive and the disease is present, the test result is a true positive. If the test result is positive but the disease is absent, the test yields a false-positive result. When the test result is negative and the disease is absent, the test result is a true negative. Finally, if the test result is negative but the disease is present, the test result is a false negative. Counting the number of true-positive, false-positive, true-negative, and false-positive results, when examining a test against a gold standard, helps define characteristics of the test, such as its sensitivity, specificity, false-negative rate, false-positive rate, predictive value, and likelihood ratio.

Sensitivity (also known as the *true-positive rate*) is defined as the proportion of patients with positive test results among all patients with the disease. For example, one might examine the DST results of patients with and without melancholic depression. Here, clinical diagnosis of melancholia is the gold standard. If there are 25 melancholic patients—20 with positive DST results and 5 with negative DST results—the sensitivity of the DST in this population is 20/25, or 80%.

Specificity (also known as the *true-negative rate*) is defined as the proportion of subjects with negative test results among those who do not have the disease. Let us suppose that there are 50 patients without melancholic depression. If 35 patients have negative DST results and 15 patients have positive DST results, the specificity of the DST in this population is 35/50, or 70%.

False-negative rate is defined as the proportion of patients with negative test results among all patients with the disease. The numbers from the sensitivity calculation can be used as an example. Five of the 25 melancholic patients have negative DST results, and 20 of the 25 melancholic patients have positive DST results. Thus, the false-negative rate is 5/25, or 20%. Note that the false-negative rate equals 1 minus the sensitivity.

False-positive rate is defined as the proportion of subjects with positive test results among those who do not have the disease. If numbers from the specificity calculation are used, 35 of 50 nonmelancholic patients have negative DST results, and 15 of 50 have positive results. The false-positive rate is 15/50, or 30%. Note that the false-positive rate equals 1 minus the specificity.

TABLE 4–1. Characteristics of a binary diagnostic test for a disease with an established gold standard diagnosis

Laboratory test results	Disease present	Gold standard test result	
		Disease absent	**Row total**
Positive	Number of TPs	Number of FPs	TPs+FPs
Negative	Number of FNs	Number of TNs	FNs+TNs
Total	TPs+FNs	FPs+TNs	Total number of subjects

Note. FN=false negative; FP=false positive; TN=true negative; TP=true positive.

Positive predictive value is defined as the proportion of patients with diseases who have positive test results among all patients with positive test results: if 20 melancholic patients and 15 nonmelancholic patients have positive DST results, a total of 35 patients have positive DST results. The positive predictive value is 20/35, or 57.1%.

Negative predictive value is defined as the proportion of patients without diseases who have negative test results among all patients with negative results. If DST results are negative in the case of 5 melancholic patients and 35 nonmelancholic patients, there are 40 patients with negative DST results. The negative predictive value is therefore 35/40, or 87.5%.

The *likelihood ratio* (LR) is the probability of having a given test result among patients with the disease, divided by the probability of having that same test result among patients without the disease. For a given test, there are two LRs: one for the finding of a positive result (LR+) and one for the finding of a negative result (LR–). Thus:

$$LR+ = \frac{\text{Probability of a positive test result among patients with disease}}{\text{Probability of a positive test result among patients without disease}} = \frac{\text{Sensitivity}}{1 - \text{Specificity}}$$

$$LR- = \frac{\text{Probability of a negative test result among patients with disease}}{\text{Probability of a negative test result among patients without disease}} = \frac{1 - \text{Sensitivity}}{\text{Specificity}}$$

The higher the likelihood ratio, the better the discriminating ability of the test. This index is also called the *odds ratio*. For example, because the sensitivity of the DST is 80% and the specificity is 70%, the LR for a positive test result is $0.8/(1-0.70)=2.67$. This indicates that the odds are 2.67 to 1 in favor of the diagnosis when the DST result is positive.

The indexes just discussed are first determined by comparing test results from two defined populations (e.g., patients with the disease and patients without the disease). However, when a test is used in a clinical setting, the story is different. The clinician wants to know whether a patient with a positive test result has the disease and whether a negative test result signifies the absence of disease. Analysis of a test result in terms of its ability to predict the presence or absence of disease in a given patient is called *operational analysis*.

Operational Level

At the operational level, the performance of the test is analyzed in reference to the clinical situation. *Operational analysis* refers to a test's performance in actual practice. Several factors can influence the predictive value of a test result. The prevalence of disease is particularly important, and this aspect of the operational analysis of a test is the one that has been best described. *Prevalence* refers to the frequency of a disease in the population being studied in a given clinical setting. If the proportion of patients with the index disease is altered, the numbers of true-positive, false-positive, false-negative, and true-negative results will be altered (see Table 4–1). In other words, predictive value changes with the prevalence of a disease in a population.

It is possible to estimate the probability that a patient will have a particular disease if one knows the prevalence of the disease and the sensitivity and specificity of the test for the population of patients being tested. The relationship between the predictive value of a positive test result and the prevalence is expressed as follows:

$$\text{Probability of disease if a positive test result} = \frac{\text{Prevalence} \times \text{Sensitivity}}{(\text{Prevalence})(\text{Sensitivity}) + (1 - \text{Prevalence})(1 - \text{Specificity})}$$

This formula is based on Bayes' theorem. (For a derivation of this formula, see Galen and Gambino [1975].) Basically, Bayes' theorem allows one to use a test to predict the presence of a disease in a given situation (i.e., the probability that a patient has a disease), provided the following are known: the prevalence of the disease, the probability of a given test result if the patient has the disease, and the probability of a given test result if the patient does not have the disease. By varying the prevalence of the disease, one can calculate, using this formula, a range of predictive values of a positive test result for a test with a given sensitivity and specificity.

Similarly, one can determine the probability that a patient has a disease when the test result is negative:

$$\text{Probability of disease if a negative test result} = \frac{\text{Prevalence} \times (1 - \text{Sensitivity})}{(\text{Prevalence})(1 - \text{Sensitivity}) + (1 - \text{Prevalence})(\text{Specificity})}$$

A number of clinical factors can affect the operational characteristics of a test. The prevalence of a disease may differ across cultures and ethnic groups. Dementia is a good example of a condition with variable prevalence across cultures and ethnicities (see "Alzheimer's Disease as a Model for Diagnostic Testing in Neuropsychiatry"). Ethnic or cultural group membership can influence testing in other ways as well. In examining genetic testing for a particular disorder, one finds that the distribution of allele frequencies often varies by race or cultural group.

Another important factor, often not discussed, is the nature of the contrasted population without the disease. For example, consider the use of the DST (with only one sample being measured at 8:00 A.M. the next day) in the diagnosis of Cushing's syndrome. The test identifies 98% of patients with Cushing's syndrome (Crapo 1979), 1% of healthy subjects (Crapo 1979), and about 51% of patients with endogenous depression (Kasper and Beckmann 1983). If the prevalence of Cushing's syndrome in a population is 50% and the prevalence of depression is 50%, the predictive value of the test for Cushing's syndrome is 65.71%. However, if the prevalence of Cushing's syndrome is 50% and the rest of the population is physically healthy, the predictive value is 99%. Therefore, the predictive value of a positive test or of a negative test depends not only on the number of patients with disease A but also on the number of patients with disease B and the number of patients with disease C.

Medical Decision–Making Level

At the medical decision–making level, the principles of decision analysis are used to assess the clinical utility of a test. Decision analysis is a systematic, explicit, and quantitative approach to making decisions under conditions of uncertainty (Raiffa 1968). There are two aspects to decision making and decision analysis. One aspect, which is prescriptive, deals with the mathematical approaches to making better decisions. The other aspect is psychological and concerns how people make decisions (Elstein et al. 1978). The prescriptive mathematical approach to decision making has been used in clinical situations. However, few attempts have been made to integrate the psychological decision theory with the mathematical approach.

The mathematical approach has been used in evaluating the utility of a test, interpreting a test, and ordering a test. One first estimates the expected utility of the test. The *expected utility* is the difference between the benefits and the costs of the test. *Cost* in this case refers to harm that may come from performing the test, such as financial costs or adverse health effects. It is assumed that if the test is to be of any use, the expected utility of choosing to order a test for a given disease must be greater than the expected utility of alternatives to ordering the test.

This leads to the next key question: When does one order a test? The concept of threshold analysis as elucidated by Pauker and Kassirer (1980) is useful for understanding when to order a test. The authors outlined two thresholds—a "testing" threshold and a "test treatment" threshold—for problems that can be reduced to three choices: treat, withhold treatment, or test and then decide on the treatment. The decision regarding the three choices is based on the probability of disease and the calculated thresholds. If the probability of disease is below the testing threshold, no treatment is given. If the probability of disease is above the test treatment threshold, treatment is given without testing. The test is ordered only if the probability is between the two thresholds. The thresholds are the points of indifference between the two decision options (i.e., the points where both options are equal). The testing threshold is the probability of disease where the expected utility of not treating is the same as the expected utility of testing followed by a treatment decision. The test treatment threshold is the probability of disease where the expected utility of treating is the same as the expected utility of testing followed by a treatment decision. By using the threshold approach, one concludes that

- the cost of the test must be lower than the risk of treatment;
- the higher the cost of the test, the lower the range of the "testing window";
- slight increases in the risk-to-benefit ratio—when that ratio falls between 0 and 1—greatly increase the testing treatment threshold;
- increasing test sensitivity increases the range of the testing window;
- increasing test specificity increases the range of the testing window;
- if the risk of testing is low, the substantial inaccuracies of testing can be tolerated;
- if the test is sufficiently accurate, substantial risks might be tolerated; and
- if the probability of disease is such that the test does not alter the therapeutic decision, the testing is superfluous and adds to the cost of patient care.

So far, we have discussed tests in terms of their utility in therapeutic decision–making. Sometimes, however, tests are ordered not for the purpose of altering a therapeutic decision but for prognostic purposes. Even in these instances, the same approach might be useful. Sometimes the test is ordered not for aiding a therapeutic decision but merely to increase or decrease the physician's suspicion about the diagnosis. The explicit approaches described are often considered by a clinician, albeit in an implicit manner (Weinstein et al. 1980). However, clinicians tend to poorly revise their probability estimates of diseases on the basis of test results. Because it makes explicit those factors that go into a decision, the decision-making analytical approach can help the clinician. By following many of the principles discussed in this section ("General Principles of Diagnostic Testing"), the clinician can make better use of diagnostic tests.

Summary of General Principles of Diagnostic Testing

We have described several levels at which tests can be analyzed. Currently, most tests are evaluated only at the analytical and diagnostic performance levels. Few tests are evaluated at the operational and medical decision–making levels, because of the difficulties associated with such evaluations.

At the analytical level, a test must be reasonably specific, sensitive, accurate, and precise if it is to provide meaningful information. At the diagnostic level, the test will provide meaningful information only if the test has both high sensitivity and high specificity and the LR is greater than 1.

At the operational level, disease prevalence and characteristics of the contrasted population alter predictive value, sensitivity, and specificity. For a test to be considered useful at the operational level, it must provide meaningful information in clinical situations. At the medical decision–making level, the test is useful only if 1) the risk of the test is lower than the risk of the treatment (or no treatment) and 2) the test result alters the probability of disease to the extent that the therapeutic decision is changed. In addition, the decision-making level gives a perspective on when to order a test.

We believe that an understanding of these principles is necessary for evaluating and interpreting laboratory tests. In the next sections, we apply these principles to and examine the diagnostic issues in AD, and we then discuss the role of neuroimaging from a standpoint of diagnosis, using the example of major depression associated with cerebrovascular disease.

Alzheimer's Disease as a Model for Diagnostic Testing in Neuropsychiatry

At present, AD is perhaps the most appropriate disease model for shedding light on the issue of diagnostic testing.

Several genetic mutations are associated with development of AD, particularly familial AD. Examples include mutations in the presenilin 1, presenilin 2, and amyloid precursor protein genes (Plassman and Breitner 1997). When symptoms of dementia are present, mutations in any of these genes confirms the diagnosis. Therefore, tests for such mutations are pathognomonic tests and likely belong in psychiatric diagnostic systems. One could make a strong case for expanding the Alzheimer's disease diagnoses in DSM to include subtypes or modifiers such as "with mutation in the presenilin 1 gene."

But not all genetic testing is pathognomonic, and this is certainly the case in AD. Apolipoprotein E (apo E), the polymorphic lipid transport protein found in the brain, has three allelic forms: ε2, ε3, and ε4. Each allele codes for a different form of apo E protein. The finding of an association between the ε4 allele and late-onset familial and sporadic AD (Saunders et al. 1993b) led to the creation of a commercial laboratory test for apo E genotype. When a diagnosis of dementia has been made, the presence of an apo E ε4 allele greatly increases the likelihood that the patient has AD, particularly if he or she is an ε4 homozygote (i.e., carries two ε4 alleles). Apo E genotyping is thus an example of a surrogate test.

But what is the relationship between apo E genotype and AD? When should this test be used? A 1997 National Institutes of Health consensus panel statement called for more investigation of the utility of apo E genetic testing in patients with dementia (Post et al. 1997). Despite the tentative tone and lack of a full endorsement, apo E genotype testing is now beginning to be used by clinicians with greater frequency as part of the workup of suspected AD. The public has also become aware of this "Alzheimer's test." We have received requests for testing from asymptomatic relatives (some in their 30s and 40s) of patients with AD.

Let us begin by examining the test for apo E genotype in light of the principles discussed in "General Principles of Diagnostic Testing."

At an analytical level, the test is very powerful, with very high accuracy and precision. One can count on a given test result correctly identifying a patient's apo E genotype.

At the level of diagnostic performance, apo E genotype testing has been well studied using autopsy-proven AD as a gold standard. Estimates of the test's sensitivity range from 65% to 83%, and its specificity ranges from 60% to 83% (Jobst et al. 1998; Mayeux et al. 1998; Saunders et al. 1996; Welsh-Bohmer et al. 1997). Positive predictive value has been reported to be very high—greater than 97% (Roses and Saunders 1997). Thus, the test performs well at the diagnostic performance level.

At the operational level, one must consider how the test performs in different clinical populations. It is at this level of consideration that the relationship between apo E genotype and occurrence of AD becomes more complex. Apo E allele frequencies differ among ethnic and racial groups, and these differences must be taken into account. In China and Japan, for example, the frequency of the ε4 allele is smaller in the general population, although an increased ε4 allele frequency associated with AD has been demonstrated (Dai et al. 1994; Hong et al. 1996; Kawamata et al. 1994; Mak et al. 1996; Nunomura et al. 1996; Okuizumi et al. 1994; Ueki et al. 1993). Unfortunately, few data are available on the distribution of alleles among African-American, Hispanic, and other racial and ethnic groups (Hendrie et al. 1995; Osuntokun et al. 1995; Saunders et al. 1993a; Tang et al. 1996).

Another consideration at the operational level is variations in the prevalence of AD and other dementias among diverse races and cultures. Estimates of dementia prevalence vary widely (Breitner et al. 1999), and such estimates are dependent on both the actual prevalence of dementia and the methods used to ascertain the prevalence, which inevitably have limitations and are not standardized across studies. Thus, for a given clinical situation, the ability to predict the probability of disease in a particular patient is limited because one cannot be precise about the prevalence of disease in the population of which the patient is a member.

One final concern regarding apo E genotype testing at the operational level relates to the association between the ε4 allele and other forms of dementia, particularly vascular dementia. In several samples around the world, an increase in the ε4 allele has been demonstrated in patients with vascular dementia (Chapman et al. 1998; Ji et al. 1998; Kalman et al. 1998; Slooter et al. 1997). Here again, one must address the issue of prevalence. What is the true prevalence of vascular dementia in a given population, and what are the methodological limitations in determining prevalence? The differential diagnosis of AD and vascular dementia is often difficult, particularly in the large population studies used to estimate dementia prevalence (Breitner et al. 1999).

At the level of medical decision–making, apo E genotype testing raises several important issues. In the section titled "Medical Decision–Making Level," we indicated that if a test is to be of any use, the expected utility of the test must be greater than the expected utility of alternatives to the test. The expected utility of apo E genotype testing is of the difference between the benefits and the costs associated with testing. Many authors have argued that the main benefit is that an accurate diagnosis can be made in patients with symptoms of dementia, without the need for ancillary and expensive tests, including neuroimaging.

The costs related to the test are more complex. At present, the cost of the test is several hundred dollars. There is also a social cost: regardless of the result of the test, the patient may be denied health or life insurance when a prospective insurer learns that such a test has been ordered. A positive test result will likely disqualify the patient for long-term care insurance. Other ethical issues stem from the larger concern about genetic testing: What does the presence of one or two ε4 alleles in the patient mean for the patient's son and sister? Should they be tested? How will that affect their insurability, let alone their psyches? Is it, in fact, a benefit that family members know the genotype? These difficult issues led a 1997 consensus panel to conclude that routine apo E genotype testing in patients with dementia may prove useful but requires further investigation, and that in nearly all cases, genetic testing in asymptomatic individuals is unwarranted (Post et al. 1997). In clinical practice, decisions about testing vary widely and are driven by physician experience with testing, practice patterns, ethical concerns about testing, patient and family insistence on testing, cost, and other factors that affect the perceived utility of the test.

Apolipoprotein E Genotype Testing: Implications for Revising the Diagnostic Classification System

What implications does apo E genotype testing have for the diagnostic classification of dementia? Six criteria (A through F) for dementia of the Alzheimer's type are listed in DSM-IV-TR. Should a criterion G be added—namely, presence of at least one apo E ε4 allele? If it is definitely decided that if a patient with dementia is an ε4 homozygote, he or she must have AD, perhaps the new criteria should be simplified to two criteria: criterion A (meets criteria for dementia) and criterion B (presence of two apo E ε4 alleles). But what about the patient with one ε4 allele or the patient with two ε4 alleles who has had a stroke?

Perhaps the issue of including apo E testing within a diagnostic criteria set is complicated by so many possible permutations that some other strategy to account for it is needed. For example, in keeping with the multiaxial system, the addition of an Axis VI, "Supporting Laboratory Data," may be warranted. Then such data could be subclassified as follows: "confirmatory of diagnosis" (e.g., test results indicating elevated thyroid function, supporting an Axis I diagnosis of anxiety disorder due to hyperthyroidism), "supportive of diagnosis" (e.g., positive DST results for diagnosis of melancholic major depression), or "rules out other diagnoses" (e.g., normal magnetic resonance image of the brain in the diagnosis of AD). Here, apo E genotype testing might fall into any of the three Axis VI categories. The condition of a patient who has a classic presentation of AD, a family history of AD, and no comorbid medical conditions and who is an ε4 homozygote might be given a C ("confirmatory of diagnosis") code, indicating apo E ε4 homozygosity. A patient with dementia who has one ε4 allele, hypertension, and white matter changes on magnetic resonance images and who otherwise appears to have AD might be given an Axis VI S ("supportive of diagnosis") code. A 50-year-old patient with profound behavioral disturbance, cognitive impairment, and Pick's disease might have his/her apo E genotype ε3/ε3 listed as an R code ("rules out other diagnoses") under Axis VI. Conditions of patients with no supporting laboratory data would have an N code ("none").

Inclusion of laboratory results within diagnostic criteria, or expansion of the multiaxial system, may not suffice. Now that the Decade of the Brain ("The Neuroanatomical Basis of Psychopathology" 1994) is concluded, should not the groundwork be laid, within a new diagnostic system, for the flood of biological advances to come? For example, psychiatric diagnoses could be simply divided into broad groups such as mood, anxiety, or cogni-

tive disorders, and the groups could then be subdivided according to biological data. This approach would eliminate the need for tedious counting
of symptoms (Does she have four or five depressive symptoms?) and meeting of criteria (Does his level of disorientation really cause him serious social dysfunction?). One could simply say, "This patient has prominent
mood symptoms; with these biological features, she therefore has major depression" or "This patient has a cognitive syndrome and apo E genotype
ε4/ε4. Therefore, he has Alzheimer's disease."

Clearly, psychiatrists' understanding of the biological underpinnings
of mental illness has not progressed to the point where a given disease is
associated with a clear laboratory marker. Even if that were the case, moving away from a nomenclature that is, at least in part, symptom based may
not be advisable. Symptom clusters, along with modifying criteria such as
duration of symptoms, have helped identify distinct and clinically meaningful diagnoses, such as major depression and dysthymia.

We favor a system that allows for the inclusion of biological markers as
they emerge. The field in which such discoveries are most likely to be made
is human genetics. With the advancement of the Human Genome Project,
it is inevitable that the genetic underpinnings of many psychiatric disorders
will become more evident. As Roses (1998) indicated, complex diseases
such as bipolar disorder and schizophrenia likely have associated sets of
susceptibility genes, and research is ongoing to identify those genes. Thus,
we favor not a search for a pathognomonic genetic test (which would sim-
plify nomenclature) but incorporation of a variety of symptom-based and
genetics-based criteria in future nosological systems.

One of the main problems with psychiatric genetics is balancing the
geneticist's need for diagnostic rigor (Is the illness present or not?) with the
clinician's observation that there are subclinical forms of disease. This is
particularly true in affective and anxiety disorders, which include severe
forms of bipolar disorder and panic as well as mild generalized anxiety and
depressive or anxious personality traits. This breadth of symptoms calls for
a precise symptom-based classification system that will allow clinical researchers and basic scientists to communicate with each other.

Neuroimaging and Psychiatric Diagnosis

Advances in technology have enabled neuroimaging research on psychiatric disorders to flourish in the past decade. Such studies involve structural
imaging using computed tomography and magnetic resonance imaging
(MRI), as well as functional imaging that employs positron emission tomography, functional MRI, magnetic resonance spectroscopy, and single

photon emission computed tomography. There is a growing consensus that major depression occurring in the context of cerebrovascular disease may be a distinct diagnostic subtype of mood disorder. Known as vascular depression, this condition usually affects older individuals with risk factors for cerebrovascular disease (Alexopoulos et al. 1997a). Characteristic features are apathy, psychomotor retardation, cognitive impairment, functional disability, and lack of family history of mood disorders (Krishnan et al. 1995, 1997). Criteria sets for vascular depression have been proposed (Alexopoulos et al. 1997b; Steffens and Krishnan 1998); vascular changes (usually in subcortical white and gray matter) demonstrated by neuroimaging have been suggested as a possible diagnostic feature. Research is needed on how well computed tomography or MRI performs in terms of the four levels of evaluation that we have discussed. In addition, it is unclear which patients may need a neuroimaging study. However, several studies have shown that consequences of severe cerebrovascular disease in the context of major depression may include poor response to treatment (Simpson et al. 1997; Steffens et al. 2001), functional impairment (Steffens et al. 2002), and increased risk of dementia (Steffens et al. 2000). Thus, it may be very important in future mood disorder diagnostic schemes to account for the presence of cerebrovascular disease. In the context of our discussion on apo E genotype testing, one could easily imagine a diagnostic system in which pertinent neuroimaging findings are placed on an Axis VI.

Summary

Where will laboratory testing fit in the new diagnostic system? Should it be restricted to disorders with known or suspected biological markers (i.e., embedded within the diagnosis), or should the possibility that testing may be instructive for all diagnoses be left open (i.e., should an Axis VI be created)? To answer these questions, we return to our apo E genotyping example. It is necessary to determine what kind of evidence or performance characteristics would be needed to add apo E ε4 as a requirement for a diagnostic criterion. Adding that requirement to the current diagnostic system would mean that all patients with AD would need to be homozygous (or at least heterozygous) for apo E ε4, something that will never occur. Given that problem, there are at least two possibilities: 1) The concept of AD as a uniform entity is incorrect, and a number of different actual etiologies for an AD-like dementia will inevitably be discovered, each of which will have its own criteria set, including a specific biological marker. The level of evidence required for each diagnosis will then need to be determined. 2) AD could remain a single diagnostic entity with several etiological subtypes, more than one of which could apply. Here, the laboratory test criterion would be embedded in the subtype (e.g., apo E type: if the patient is homozygous for apo E ε4, or if the patient is heterozygous for apo E ε4 and has a positive family history for Alzheimer's dementia).

One alternative to embedding laboratory testing within certain criteria is increasing the number of axes to six. This would necessitate that testing be considered for all patients being evaluated, at all times; this is the point of the multiaxial system. The advantage of this approach is that it retains the multiaxial system while allowing for inclusion of laboratory data. There are at least a few disadvantages. First, the approach leaves testing up to the clinician; treatment guidelines would need to be established for when to order tests. Guidelines would also need to specify how to code a given test result on Axis VI. Development and adoption of guidelines for ordering tests and completing Axis VI might become so complicated that a diagnostic workup could not be easily performed, because of the time involved, the expense, or the lack of access to testing. A second disadvantage to the Axis VI approach is that it might not fully address biological advances. For instance, absolutely pathognomonic tests might be developed (e.g., if the patient has this gene or set of genes and has any mood symptoms, he or she has bipolar disorder), leaving biological markers in asymptomatic patients unaddressed. One example is the gene for Huntington's disease. Unaffected children of patients with the disease can undergo the test. Such testing is important to the children for many reasons; for example, results will figure into their decisions about having children. How should the conditions of such patients be classified? Will an Axis VI diagnosis in an asymptomatic individual prevent him or her from obtaining health or life insurance? These are difficult questions that must be faced as consideration is given regarding how to include testing, especially genetic testing, in psychiatric classification schemes.

We favor an approach that both retains symptom-based criteria and is flexible enough to accommodate (or even anticipate) biological discoveries as they emerge. Adding an Axis VI to DSM-V would accomplish this goal, but such an addition must be carefully considered beforehand. Clinicians, ethicists, and researchers will need to weigh in on the proper approach for promoting effective clinical care, advancing research, and providing ethical safeguards for individual patients and for society.

References

Alexopoulos GS, Meyers BS, Young RC, et al: Clinically defined vascular depression. Am J Psychiatry 154:562–565, 1997a

Alexopoulos GS, Meyers BS, Young RC, et al: 'Vascular depression' hypothesis. Arch Gen Psychiatry 54:915–922, 1997b

American Psychiatric Association: Diagnostic and Statistical Manual of Mental Disorders, 4th Edition, Text Revision. Washington, DC, American Psychiatric Association, 2000

Breitner JC, Wyse BW, Anthony JC, et al: APOE-epsilon4 count predicts age when prevalence of AD increases, then declines: the Cache County Study. Neurology 53:321–331, 1999

Chapman J, Wang N, Treves TA, et al: ACE, MTHFR, factor V Leiden, and APOE polymorphisms in patients with vascular and Alzheimer's dementia. Stroke 29:1401–1404, 1998

Crapo L: Cushing's syndrome: a review of diagnostic tests. Metabolism 28:955–977, 1979

Cruts M, Hendriks L, Van Broeckhoven C: The presenilin genes: a new gene family involved in Alzheimer disease pathology. Hum Mol Genet 5 (Spec No):1449–1455, 1996

Dai XY, Nanko S, Hattori M, et al: Association of apolipoprotein E4 with sporadic Alzheimer's disease is more pronounced in early onset type. Neurosci Lett 175:74–76, 1994

Elstein AS, Shulman LS, Sprafka SA: Medical Problem Solving: An Analysis of Clinical Reasoning. Cambridge, MA, Harvard University Press, 1978

Feinstein AR: Clinical Biostatistics. St. Louis, MO, Mosby, 1977

Galen RS: Selection of appropriate laboratory tests, in Clinician and Chemist. Edited by Young DS, Nipper H, Uddin D, et al. Washington, DC, American Association for Clinical Chemistry, 1982, pp 69–105

Galen RS, Gambino SR: Beyond Normality: The Predictive Value and Efficiency of Medical Diagnoses. New York, Wiley, 1975

Hendrie HC, Hall KS, Hui S, et al: Apolipoprotein E genotypes and Alzheimer's disease in a community study of elderly African Americans. Ann Neurol 37:118–120, 1995

Hong CJ, Liu TY, Liu HC, et al: Epsilon 4 allele of apolipoprotein E increases risk of Alzheimer's disease in a Chinese population. Neurology 46:1749–1751, 1996

Ji Y, Urakami K, Adachi Y, et al: Apolipoprotein E polymorphism in patients with Alzheimer's disease, vascular dementia and ischemic cerebrovascular disease. Dement Geriatr Cogn Disord 9:243–245, 1998

Jobst KA, Barnetson LP, Shepstone BJ: Accurate prediction of histologically confirmed Alzheimer's disease and the differential diagnosis of dementia: the use of NINCDS-ADRDA and DSM-III-R criteria, SPECT, X-ray CT, and Apo E4 in medial temporal lobe dementias. Oxford Project to Investigate Memory and Aging. Int Psychogeriatr 10:271–302, 1998

Kalman J, Juhasz A, Csaszar A, et al: Increased apolipoprotein E4 allele frequency is associated with vascular dementia in the Hungarian population. Acta Neurol Scand 98:166–168, 1998

Kasper S, Beckmann M: Dexamethasone suppression tests in a pluridiagnostic approach: its relationship to psychopathological and clinical variables. Acta Psychiatr Scand 68:31–37, 1983

Kawamata J, Tanaka S, Shimohama S, et al: Apolipoprotein E polymorphism in Japanese patients with Alzheimer's disease or vascular dementia. Neurol Neurosurg Psychiatry 57:1414–1416, 1994

Krishnan KR, Davidson JR, Rayasam K, et al: Diagnostic utility of the dexamethasone suppression test. Biol Psychiatry 22:618–628, 1987

Krishnan KR, Hays JC, Tupler LA, et al: Clinical and phenomenological comparisons of late-onset and early-onset depression. Am J Psychiatry 152:785–788, 1995

Krishnan KR, Hays JC, Blazer DG: MRI-defined vascular depression. Am J Psychiatry 154:497–501, 1997

Mak YT, Chiu H, Woo J, et al: Apolipoprotein E genotype and Alzheimer's disease in Hong Kong elderly Chinese. Neurology 46:146–149, 1996

Mayeux R, Saunders AM, Shea S, et al: Utility of the apolipoprotein E genotype in the diagnosis of Alzheimer's disease. Alzheimer's Disease Centers Consortium on Apolipoprotein E and Alzheimer's Disease. N Engl J Med 338:506–511, 1998

The Neuroanatomical Basis of Psychopathology: The Decade of the Brain. 49th Annual Convention and Scientific Program of the Society of Biological Psychiatry. Philadelphia, Pennsylvania, May 18–22, 1994. Abstracts. Biol Psychiatry 35:579–756, 1994

Nunomura A, Chiba S, Eto M, et al: Apolipoprotein E polymorphism and susceptibility to early and late-onset sporadic Alzheimer's disease in Hokkaido, the northern part of Japan. Neurosci Lett 206:17–20, 1996

Okuizumi K, Onodera O, Tanaka H, et al: ApoE-epsilon 4 and early onset Alzheimer's. Nat Genet 7:10–11, 1994

Osuntokun BO, Sahota A, Ogunniyi AO, et al: Lack of an association between apolipoprotein E epsilon 4 and Alzheimer's disease in elderly Nigerians. Ann Neurol 38:463–465, 1995

Pauker SG, Kassirer JP: The threshold approach to clinical decision making. N Engl J Med 302:1109–1117, 1980

Plassman BL, Breitner JCS: The genetics of dementia in late life. Psychiatr Clin North Am 20:59–76, 1997

Post SG, Whitehouse PJ, Binstock RH, et al: The clinical introduction of genetic testing for Alzheimer disease: an ethical perspective. JAMA 277:832–836, 1997

Raiffa H: Decision Analysis: Introductory Lectures on Choices Under Uncertainty. Reading, MA, Addison-Wesley, 1968

Ransahoff D, Feinstein AR: Problems of spectrum and bias in evaluating the efficacy of diagnostic tests. N Engl J Med 299:926–929, 1978

Roses AD: Alzheimer diseases: a model of gene mutations and susceptibility polymorphisms for complex psychiatric diseases. Am J Med Genet 81:49–57, 1998

Roses AD, Saunders AM: Apolipoprotein E genotyping as a diagnostic adjunct for Alzheimer's disease. Int Psychogeriatr 9 (suppl 1):277–288, 1997

Saunders AM, Schmader K, Breitner JC, et al: Apolipoprotein E epsilon 4 allele distributions in late-onset Alzheimer's disease and in other amyloid-forming diseases. Lancet 342:710–711, 1993a

Saunders AM, Strittmatter WJ, Schmechel D, et al: Association of apolipoprotein E allele epsilon 4 with late-onset familial and sporadic Alzheimer's disease. Neurology 43:1467–1472, 1993b

Saunders AM, Hulette O, Welsh-Bohmer KA, et al: Specificity, sensitivity, and predictive value of apolipoprotein-E genotyping for sporadic Alzheimer's disease. Lancet 348:90–93, 1996

Simpson SW, Jackson A, Baldwin RC, et al: 1997 IPA/Bayer Research Awards in Psychogeriatrics. Subcortical hyperintensities in late-life depression: acute response to treatment and neuropsychological impairment. Int Psychogeriatr 9:257–275, 1997

Slooter AJ, Tang MX, van Duijn CM, et al: Apolipoprotein E epsilon4 and the risk of dementia with stroke: a population-based investigation. JAMA 277:818–821, 1997

Steffens DC, Krishnan KR: Structural neuroimaging and mood disorders: recent findings, implications for classification, and future directions. Biol Psychiatry 43:705–712, 1998

Steffens DC, MacFall JR, Payne ME, et al: Grey-matter lesions and dementia. Lancet 356:1686–1687, 2000

Steffens DC, Conway CR, Dombeck CB, et al: Severity of subcortical gray matter hyperintensity predicts ECT response in geriatric depression. J ECT 17:45–49, 2001

Steffens DC, Bosworth HB, Provenzale JM, et al: Subcortical white matter lesions and functional impairment in geriatric depression. Depress Anxiety 15:23–28, 2002

Tang MX, Maestre G, Tsai WY, et al: Relative risk of Alzheimer disease and age-at-onset distributions, based on APOE genotypes among elderly African Americans, Caucasians, and Hispanics in New York City. Am J Hum Genet 58:574–584, 1996

Ueki A, Kawano M, Namba Y, et al: A high frequency of apolipoprotein E4 isoprotein in Japanese patients with late-onset nonfamilial Alzheimer's disease. Neurosci Lett 163:166–168, 1993

Weinstein MC, Fineberg HV, Elstein AS, et al: Clinical Decision Analysis. Philadelphia, PA, WB Saunders, 1980

Welsh-Bohmer KA, Gearing M, Saunders AM, et al: Apolipoprotein E genotypes in a neuropathological series from the Consortium to Establish a Registry for Alzheimer's Disease. Ann Neurol 42:319–325, 1997

CHAPTER 5

Insights From Neuroscience for the Concept of Schizotaxia and the Diagnosis of Schizophrenia

Ming T. Tsuang, M.D., Ph.D., D.Sc., F.R.C.Psych.,
William S. Stone, Ph.D., Sarah I. Tarbox, B.A.,
Stephen V. Faraone, Ph.D.

Psychiatric diagnosis and classification have progressed substantially since the seminal observations of Kraepelin and Bleuler provided the basis for classification systems in the middle of the twentieth century. The ambiguous diagnostic definitions that characterized DSM-I (American Psychiatric Association 1952) and DSM-II (American Psychiatric Association 1968) were replaced by more reliable criteria in DSM-III (American Psychiatric Association 1980) and later editions of the manual (Blashfield 1984). Because the newer criteria were more precise than earlier formulations and were based on symptoms rather than etiological theory, they allowed for more accurate and uniform estimates of the rates of disorders around the world. Despite the important advances in the evolution of DSM, the diagnostic criteria for mental disorders have remained, in some ways, relatively unchanged since their inception. This latter point is demonstrated clearly by the continued reliance on clinical symptoms for psychiatric diagnosis.

There is little question that recent (DSM-III and later) diagnostic criteria have made diagnoses more reliable and, to some extent, more valid. This progress raises the issue of whether still more improvement can be

Preparation of this chapter was supported in part by National Institute of Mental Health grants 1 R01 MH4187901, 5 UO1 MH4631802, R25 MH60485, and 1 R37 MH4351801 (Dr. Tsuang and the Department of Veterans Affairs Medical Research Service, Health Services Research and Development Service, and Cooperative Studies Programs); a National Alliance for Research on Schizophrenia and Depression (NARSAD) Distinguished Investigator Award (Dr. Tsuang); and a NARSAD Young Investigator Award (Dr. Stone).

made. Ultimately, the conceptualization of most mental disorders—and, consequently, the diagnostic criteria used to identify them—will incorporate an understanding of their neurobiological etiologies. This would seem to be a natural development, especially given the progress made in neuroscience and genetics in just the last 10 years. Yet current diagnostic criteria for psychiatric conditions do not include neurobiological signs or symptoms. The main reason for this has been the inability to establish the usefulness of such signs and symptoms empirically.

In light of recent progress, however, it may be time to reconsider the value of neurobiological signs and symptoms. In this chapter, we review the issue, focusing on schizophrenia and related disorders. We consider representative examples of biological abnormalities in schizophrenia to assess their potential value as diagnostic markers (i.e., criteria) for these conditions. To identify abnormalities that may be relatively specific to schizophrenia, we emphasize conditions that may indicate predisposition to schizophrenia (i.e., schizotaxia) in nonpsychotic relatives of patients with schizophrenia. Directions for future investigation are then considered. We begin, however, with a discussion of the limitations of DSM-IV-TR (American Psychiatric Association 2000) diagnostic criteria for schizophrenia.

Current Boundaries of DSM Diagnostic Criteria for Schizophrenia

Stringent, narrow diagnostic criteria for disorders such as schizophrenia were needed in the 1970s and 1980s to improve the reliability of clinical diagnoses and to counteract the prevailing view that mental illnesses are myths that harm patients by stigmatizing them. Periodic revisions of the major classification systems have refined diagnoses and increased their reliability and have facilitated the adoption of empirical methods to determine which symptoms most appropriately characterize specific disorders. Because of the reliability of diagnoses in recent DSMs, the clinical characteristics of samples are more standardized across studies, and findings of these studies are thus more easily replicated. Moreover, the use of stringent diagnostic criteria laid the groundwork for studies assessing the validity of schizophrenia, and these studies have in fact demonstrated substantial concurrent and predictive validity. For example, schizophrenia can be discriminated from other disorders, shows familial loading, and predicts measures of outcome (e.g., greater functional impairment is predictive of larger numbers of recurrent episodes).

Can the classification of schizophrenia be further improved? Can the integration of current knowledge with existing conceptual classification schemes enhance psychiatrists' diagnostic abilities? In this context, at least three limitations of the current diagnostic criteria can be addressed: schizophrenia is viewed as a discrete category; the criteria are only descriptive and do not incorporate information about the etiology and pathophysiology of the disorder; and psychosis is emphasized. Each of these limitations leads to the same question: Can the reliability of the DSM-IV-TR diagnosis of schizophrenia be retained while the validity of diagnosis is improved? These points are discussed in the following three sections.

DSM-IV-TR Schizophrenia as a Discrete Category

In DSM-IV-TR, schizophrenia (like other disorders) is defined as a discrete category rather than a quantitative dimension. An implication of this approach is that schizophrenia differs qualitatively from states of health. In this view, schizophrenia begins with the onset of the symptoms listed in DSM-IV-TR. Before that time, however, the disorder cannot be diagnosed. Therefore, if the criteria for other disorders are also not met, no psychiatric diagnoses can be made. To a significant degree, making the decision hinges on whether psychotic symptoms are present.

In cases of patients with symptoms of multiple disorders, a reliance on discrete categories may lead to artificial boundary conditions and/or increased rates of comorbidity (Frances et al. 1991). For example, some individuals with schizotypal or borderline personality disorder may also meet criteria for Axis I anxiety or affective disorders when aspects of their underlying disorders might (potentially) be better explained by a dimensional view such as neuroticism. Certainly, dimensional models of psychopathology have conceptual and pragmatic limitations as well (Frances et al. 1991; Gunderson et al. 1991; Millon 1991). However, this question remains: Does a dimensional model describe more accurately than a categorical model the biological nature of schizophrenia?

Certainly a dimensional view of schizophrenia is more consistent (compared with a categorical one) with polygenic models of inheritance, which account the best for familial transmission of schizophrenia (Gottesman 1991; Tsuang et al. 1999a). The assumption of polygenic models is that multiple genes combine with one another and with environmental factors to cause schizophrenia. Because multiple genes and environmental risk factors are involved, it is possible for people to have low, moderate, or high "doses" of risk factors that predispose to schizophrenia. People with very high doses are at high risk for schizophrenia, whereas those with moderate doses may have related conditions such as schizotypal personality disorder, negative symptoms, neuropsychological impairment, or other neurobiological manifestations of the predisposition to schizophrenia (Faraone et al. 1995a). From this perspective, a dimensional model describes the range of schizophrenic illness better than does a categorical one.

In fact, a partial foundation for a dimensional view of the biological or clinical manifestations of the vulnerability to schizophrenia already exists in the research on schizotaxia, a term originally introduced by Meehl (1962) to describe the unexpressed genetic predisposition to schizophrenia. Meehl (1962) suggested that individuals with schizotaxia develop either schizotypy or schizophrenia, depending on the protection or liability afforded by environmental circumstances. He later proposed that schizotaxia need not progress into either of these more overt conditions (Meehl 1989). Given current data showing that environmental events (e.g., obstetric complications, viruses), in addition to genes, augment susceptibility to schizophrenia, Faraone et al. (2001) proposed the use of the term *schizotaxia* to indicate the premorbid, neurobiological substrate of schizophrenia.

Today, 40 years after the idea of schizotaxia was first advanced, a preponderance of evidence shows it to be a clinically meaningful condition. In fact, studies involving nonschizotypal, nonpsychotic relatives of schizophrenic patients demonstrate that schizotaxia is not merely a theoretical construct but an entity with distinct psychiatric and neurobiological features, including negative symptoms, neuropsychological impairment, and neurobiological abnormalities (Faraone et al. 2001). Tsuang et al. (1999b) described initial research criteria for schizotaxia based on at least moderate levels of negative symptoms and neuropsychological deficits in long-term verbal memory, attention, and/or executive functions (e.g., forming abstractions to solve problems).

Schizotaxia is a broader construct than schizophrenia. Our empirical studies suggest that the symptoms of schizotaxia occur in 20%–50% of first-degree relatives of schizophrenic patients (Faraone et al. 1995a, 1995b). In comparison, only about 10% of relatives become psychotic, and fewer than 10% develop schizotypal personality disorder (Battaglia and Torgersen 1996; Battaglia et al. 1995). These figures suggest that schizotaxia does not lead inevitably to schizotypal personality or schizophrenia but is, in most cases, a long-term condition. These findings lead to the question of what type of etiological model accounts best for a long-term biological vulnerability (schizotaxia) that under some circumstances results in more serious conditions (schizophrenia). These findings also suggest that the dimensional model of schizophrenia may have greater validity than the categorical model.

Dissociation of Diagnostic Criteria From Etiology and Pathophysiology

In DSM-III (and later editions of DSM), diagnostic criteria were explicitly dissociated from speculation about etiology, to prevent incorporation of etiological theories not subjected to empirical tests. At this point, however, one should not consider empirical facts about etiology as irrelevant to diagnosis. Such a view also risks a continuing disconnection of treatment from etiology. Since the introduction of antipsychotic medications, pharmacological treatments have focused on alleviating the most acute, florid symptoms of schizophrenia (i.e., those related to psychosis). Although several newer antipsychotic medications also alleviate selected negative symptoms and cognitive deficits, treatment remains symptomatic. It is not aimed at addressing specific causes of the disorder, nor is it aimed at preventing its onset.

Schizophrenia's pathophysiology is in place long before the first psychotic episode. Many researchers have sketched neurodevelopmental models of schizophrenia based on adverse genetic and environmental interactions that occur as early as the second trimester of life (see, for example, Cannon 1996; Cannon et al. 1994a; Goldman-Rakic 1995; Seidman 1990; Tsuang and Faraone 1995; Weinberger 1987, 1994, 1995; Woods 1998). If this perspective is accurate, then these events create a neurodevelopmental syndrome that includes the type of neuropsychological, neurobiological, and clinical abnormalities that characterize schizophrenic patients and their nonpsychotic relatives (Faraone et al. 2001). For reasons that are still unknown, this syndrome sometimes leads to psychosis and sometimes does not. Notably, these indicators of the syndrome are more proximal to schizophrenia's initial causes than is psychosis.

Psychosis as Sine Qua Non in Schizophrenia

Psychosis has long been considered necessary for the diagnosis of schizophrenia. But is it truly specific to schizophrenia, or is it a nonspecific indicator of severe mental illness? A variety of evidence supports the latter view. It is clear that psychosis is specific neither to schizophrenia nor even to psychiatric disorders. It occurs, for example, in neurological disease (e.g., Alzheimer's disease, Huntington's disease, schizophrenia-like psychosis of epilepsy, vascular dementia, and traumatic brain injury) and can be caused by a range of toxic substances or impaired metabolic states. Even Schneiderian first-rank symptoms, which have played such a prominent role in defining the nature of psychotic symptoms in modern diagnostic systems, are not specific to schizophrenia (Peralta and Cuesta 1998). Similarly, several recent factor-analytic studies showed that measures of psychosis in schizophrenia did not differentiate psychosis from other forms of psychopathology (Bell et al. 1998; Peralta et al. 1997; Ratakonda et al. 1998; Serretti et al. 1996). Psychotic symptoms occurring in other diagnostic groups have also been described (Crow 1998a; Monti and Stanhellini

1996), although the issue of whether types of psychotic symptoms might be specific to schizophrenia remains controversial (see, for example, Kendler et al. 1998).

Several molecular genetic studies failed to show linkage to schizophrenia on the basis of the DSM diagnosis, finding instead stronger evidence for linkage when the phenotype was broadened to include additional psychotic disorders (Maziade et al. 1997; Wildenauer et al. 1996). Other genetic studies have also added to accumulating evidence that different psychotic disorders share common elements (Wildenauer et al. 1999). Moreover, schizophrenia and affective disorders occur at increased rates in families with either schizophrenia or affective disorders (see, for example, Maier et al. 1993), and evidence for genetic linkage for both types of psychotic disorders has been obtained at similar chromosomal loci. Ginns et al. (1996), for instance, obtained evidence for linkage at 6p for bipolar disorder in Old Order Amish pedigrees, near the same chromosomal region that Maziade et al. (1997) and others identified. Similarly, the chromosome 10p region was implicated in both schizophrenia and bipolar disorder in the National Institute of Mental Health Genetics Initiative pedigrees (Faraone et al. 1998; Foroud et al. 1998; Rice et al. 1997), and regions in 13q and 18p were also implicated recently in both of these disorders (Wildenauer et al. 1999).

One rationale for the similarities among psychotic symptoms in different disorders may involve inherent pathophysiological effects of psychosis. Several lines of evidence support this possibility. One stems from observations that clinical outcomes of schizophrenia improve when treatment is obtained early in the illness (Wyatt 1995). Another involves the growing body of evidence that some patients with schizophrenia have neurobiological abnormalities, such as enlarged ventricles, loss of tissue volume, degeneration of membrane phospholipids, delayed P300 waves in event-related–potential paradigms (Knoll et al. 1998), and abnormal gamma-aminobutyric acid (GABA)–ergic neurotransmission (Keverne 1999).

Thus, similarities among psychotic symptoms in different disorders may be apparent at multiple genetic and biological levels, as well as phenomenologically. What are the implications of such similarities? Crow (1990, 1991, 1998b) proposed a continuum of psychosis that crosses diagnostic boundaries and suggested that schizophrenia, schizoaffective disorder, and affective illness exist along one or more such continua. Although he accepted the view that prototypical entities correspond to schizophrenia and affective illness, he rejected the idea that they have distinct etiologies. Instead, he hypothesized that natural variation along one or more dimensions produces the prototypical disorders. He postulated that psychotic disorders share a genetic deficit, located in the pseudoautosomal region of the sex chromosomes, and that genes related to psychosis are responsible for cerebral dominance and the localization of language.

Support for the pseudoautosomal hypothesis is weak (Collinge et al. 1991; DeLisi et al. 1994; Parfitt et al. 1991), and a psychosis gene shared by all psychotic disorders has yet to be discovered. Nevertheless, Crow's view of psychosis is intriguing. If psychosis has an etiology apart from other core symptoms of schizophrenia, DSM's diagnostic focus on psychosis in schizophrenia could be a mistake. In the hunt for the causes of schizophrenia, psychosis could be a red herring.

The foregoing discussion of common elements in psychoses is consistent with Crow's notion of a continuum of psychosis, in regard to common phenomenology and etiology. It differs from Crow's view, however, in its implications for the construct of schizophrenia. Similarities among psychotic states do not necessarily imply that the underlying disorders lie on the same continuum. An alternative view is that because psychotic states may impair functioning in a relatively global manner, and may have adverse neuropathological effects of their own, their net effect may be to emphasize superficial similarities among such disorders while obscuring more subtle, but defining, differences.

In summary, there are two problems associated with the use of psychosis as a sine qua non in schizophrenia. First, mounting evidence suggests that psychosis may be the "fever" of severe mental illness. Although psychosis is a serious problem, it is a nonspecific indicator. Second, psychosis is an end-state condition that, in comparison with other indicators, is a relatively distant consequence of schizophrenia's causes and pathophysiology. If these views are correct, the focus on psychosis may actually hinder the search for the causes of schizophrenia.

These conclusions provide support for an alternative conceptualization of schizophrenic illness, one based on the notion of schizotaxia. If this conceptualization is correct, it may be a more specific expression of the predisposition to schizophrenia than is the DSM-IV-TR diagnosis of schizophrenia. Unlike schizophrenia, schizotaxia is not masked by the florid clinical symptoms and possible neurotoxic consequences of psychosis that are seen in so many other conditions. The criteria would presumably reflect the biological and clinical alterations that occur before the advent of psychosis. If these new criteria were used, the diagnosis of schizophrenia would comprise two categories: schizotaxia and schizotaxia with psychosis (schizophrenia). This approach would be analogous to the classification of depression. In this formulation, schizotaxia with psychosis would correlate with the DSM-IV-TR view of the disorder (schizophrenia). Schizophrenia without psychosis would be equivalent to schizotaxia.

Although the formulation is reasonable, it requires that the nature and the validity of schizotaxia be demonstrated. In the next section, we consider several neurobiological abnormalities that may be related to schizotaxia.

Emerging Role for Endophenotypes in Diagnosis

Many clinical and neurobiological abnormalities that occur in patients with schizophrenia also occur in their nonpsychotic, first-degree relatives. These include eye tracking dysfunction (Levy et al. 1994), allusive thinking (Catts et al. 1993), neurological signs (Erlenmeyer-Kimling et al. 1982), biochemical abnormalities (Callicott et al. 1998), characteristic auditory evoked potentials (Friedman and Squires-Wheeler 1994), brain abnormalities revealed by neuroimaging (Seidman et al. 1997b), and neuropsychological impairment (Kremen et al. 1994). In this section, we consider a few of these abnormalities to illustrate their potential value as markers of predisposition to schizophrenia.

Genetics

Etiological Genes Involved in Schizophrenia

It has long been clear that genes play a major etiological role in the development of schizophrenia (Gottesman 1991; Tsuang et al. 1999a). The development of polygenic mathematical models to account for patterns of illness in families has been aided enormously by the continued refinement of computer programs to analyze data under a variety of etiological assumptions. This progress raises the issue of whether such models can guide molecular genetic research to discover etiological genes involved in schizophrenia. Research in this area increased significantly over the last 20 years, spurred in part by the improvement of DNA markers used to find susceptibility genes (Tsuang et al. 1999a).

Although several forms of molecular genetic analyses are available, linkage analysis, a particularly versatile procedure, might be able to explain the familial basis of schizophrenia. Linkage analysis recently provided promising evidence in the search for the origins of the disorder. Briefly, linkage analysis capitalizes on events that occur during meiosis, when chromosomes cross over and exchange segments of DNA. During this process, genes that are closer to each other are more likely to be inherited together than are genes that are farther apart. The probability of identifying a disease gene is increased if it cosegregates (i.e., is "linked") with an allele whose chromosomal location can be identified among members of a family. Linkage analysis is assessment of the probability that a marker gene and a disease gene do, in fact, cosegregate. Several factors are crucial for linkage studies to succeed, including knowledge (or presumption) of the mode of inheritance; the involvement of susceptibility genes whose effects are large enough to detect; and the accurate classification of family members as either affected or not affected by a condition caused by schizophrenia susceptibility genes.

With these considerations in mind, let us turn to the status of linkage studies of schizophrenia. Hopes were first raised in the late 1980s, when two groups reported linkage to a susceptibility gene on chromosome 5 (Bassett 1989; Sherrington et al. 1988). Unfortunately, the findings were not replicated in other studies and were eventually regarded as false-positive responses (Tsuang et al. 1999a). Over the next several years, this pattern was repeated all too often. Initial reports of linkage raised hopes that were then deflated by subsequent nonreplications. At the same time, however, more precise DNA markers were developed, and greater statistical power was obtained through large, international collaborative efforts. In the last few years, these approaches have begun to bear fruit: positive findings are finally beginning to be replicated with some regularity. The first of these replications were reported at chromosomes 6p and 8p in 1995, and recent replications were achieved at chromosomes 10p, 13q, 15q, and 22q (see Tsuang et al. 1999a). A major susceptibility locus for familial schizophrenia has been identified at chromosome 1q21-22 (Brzustowicz et al. 2000).

Pharmacogenetics and Pharmacogenomics

The underlying notion of pharmacogenetics was described more than 40 years ago (Motulsky 1957) and was based on the concept that genetic variation affects drug metabolism. That focus reflected technological advances that permitted the identification of enzymes involved in drug metabolism (such as cytochrome P450 [CYP] enzymes) and drug metabolites. In its more recent applications to psychiatry, this approach has been promising. For instance, it recently led to evidence that variants of specific cytochrome P450 enzymes (e.g., CYP 2C9, CYP 2C19, and CYP 2D6 [a variant of CYP 2D6 is also known as the sparteine-debrisoquin polymorphism]) are related to good and poor metabolism of these enzymes (see, for example, Cichon et al. 2000; Coutts and Urichuk 1999).

A question that arises in the study of psychiatric disorders particularly is how pharmacogenetics might be related to brain function. In the context of psychiatric disorders, studies that aim at a pharmacokinetic level of analysis might not be quite as useful, ultimately, as studies that focus on polymorphisms expressed in the brain. The goal of this "pharmacodynamic" approach (Cichon et al. 2000) is to identify genetically influenced variability in biological substrates that are the actual targets of psychoactive drugs. Largely because of the progress made by the Human Genome Project, human gene sequences will be available in the near future, and these sequences will also permit identification of genetic variations in those genes. The domain of potential sources of variability in response to antipsychotic medication is large. It includes the sequence of steps involved in synaptic transmission, from presynaptic mechanisms of synthesis, transport, storage, and release, to postsynaptic receptor mechanisms (including second- and third-messenger systems, subsequent postsynaptic genetic modifications, and mechanisms of degradation). Eventually, identification of such sources of variability (i.e., differential responses to medications or other pharmacological probes) may facilitate individualized treatments for schizophrenia as well as identification of subtypes of schizophrenia—or identification of nonpsychotic individuals with a predisposition for the disorder.

The ability of genetic studies to identify schizophrenia genes and schizophrenia-related conditions is still in the early stages. However, several expressions of the disorder that are intermediate between the susceptibility genes (and adverse environmental events) that caused them and the DSM clinical symptoms they ultimately give rise to are available for study. Among these endophenotypes (Gottesman 1991) are neuropsychological, neuroimaging, and psychophysiological abnormalities.

Neuropsychology

Clinical neuropsychological studies have long demonstrated dysfunctions in schizophrenia, particularly impairments in attention (Nuechterlein and Dawson 1984), executive function (Goldberg and Seidman 1991; Seidman et al. 1992), declarative and working memory (Goldman-Rakic 1991; Seidman et al. 1998b), and language and reasoning abilities (Andreasen 1979). Cognitive neuropsychological studies have also emphasized generalized deficits, without clear identification of differentially selective difficulties (Seidman et al. 1992), because schizophrenic patients perform poorly on many tasks when processing loads (i.e., resource demands) are high. Overload of information processing occurs when tasks are made more effortful through increases in short-term memory requirements, division of attention (dual-task paradigms), and increases in interference (Granholm et al. 1996; Seidman et al. 1998a). Thus, cognitive deficits are greatest when the schizophrenic patient must pay attention to more than one stimulus, divide his or her attention among stimuli, or ignore irrelevant stimuli.

In schizophrenic patients with multiple cognitive deficits and generalized performance problems, it is difficult to determine true primary cognitive deficits (Chapman and Chapman 1989). This difficulty provides an important rationale for studying such patients' close biological relatives, who are less severely affected. Moreover, studies involving such relatives rarely have to account for effects of medications or institutionalizations or for neurotoxic effects of psychosis. (With respect to the latter point, for example, earlier treatments are associated with better clinical outcomes [Wyatt 1995].) More direct evidence for biological effects of psychosis includes findings that ventricular enlargement is greater in patients with schizophrenia than in nonpsychotic patients with schizotypal personality disorder, although both groups have enlarged ventricles and sulci compared with those of control subjects, and the extent of sulcal enlargement is the same in patients with schizophrenia and nonpsychotic patients with schizotypal personality disorder (Cannon 1996; Cannon et al. 1994a).

Thus, relatives of schizophrenic patients have been studied in order to obtain potential evidence of vulnerability to the illness, identify phenotypic markers, and focus on the core pathophysiology of the disorder with fewer confounding variables than in patient studies.

Studies involving relatives clearly show a range of neuropsychological deficits (Cannon et al. 1994b; Erlenmeyer-Kimling 2000; Faraone et al. 1999a, 2001; Green et al. 1997b; Park et al. 1995). As in schizophrenia, deficits in executive functions, attention, working memory, and long-term declarative memory occur consistently (Faraone et al. 1995a, 1995b, 2001). In a 4-year follow-up study, we determined that these deficits were generally stable over time (Faraone et al. 1999a). Moreover, they tend to co-occur in relatives, but not in control subjects (Toomey et al. 1998), and they are more severe when relatives have more than one close biological relative with schizophrenia (i.e., the genetic loading is higher) (Faraone et al. 2000).

Neuroimaging

Structural Magnetic Resonance Imaging

Most magnetic resonance imaging (MRI) studies show greater volume loss in the brains of schizophrenic patients than in their nonpsychotic siblings (Sharma et al. 1998; Suddath et al. 1990), although these relatives (particularly those with schizotypal personality disorder or an especially high genetic loading for schizophrenia) may also exhibit neuroanatomical abnormalities (Sharma et al. 1998). Cannon et al. (1997), using MRI to investigate the cortex, demonstrated reduced cortical gray matter in unaffected siblings of schizophrenic patients. Keshavan et al. (1997) used structural MRI and magnetic resonance spectroscopy in a study involving offspring at risk for schizophrenia and found that adolescent offspring of patients with schizophrenia ("high-risk" offspring) had reduced left amygdala volume, enlarged third ventricle volume, and smaller overall brain volume.

These findings suggest that components of the neurobiological predisposition to schizophrenia could be expressed in relatives of schizophrenic patients as structural brain abnormalities that are independent of psychosis. In fact, volume abnormalities are evident in a variety of brain regions, including the amygdala-hippocampus region, thalamus, cerebellum, and pallidum (Seidman et al. 1997b). Similarly, in other studies involving schizophrenic patients, enlargements of the third and lateral ventricles are the most common findings.

Functional Magnetic Resonance Imaging

Fewer functional than structural MRI studies have been conducted. In one pilot study, we compared 13 never-psychotic, non–spectrum disorder relatives of schizophrenic patients and 12 matched control subjects (Seidman et al. 1997a). Relatives were significantly impaired in performing working memory tasks with interference. The most striking finding involved the different number of regions activated and the extent of regional activations (the number of voxels) in relatives compared with control subjects. Across the three tasks, relatives had a greater number of activations (significantly more activated voxels) than did control subjects. During working memory tasks and memory-plus-interference tasks, activation was more bilaterally distributed in relatives than in control subjects. Because relatives also performed worse on these cognitive tasks, these large and extraneous activations in relatives may represent 1) compensatory exertion of inefficient neural circuitry during effortful tasks and/or 2) abnormal connectivity in the circuitry required to perform these tasks.

Psychophysiology

A number of significant psychophysiological abnormalities are evident in schizophrenic patients and their nonpsychotic first-degree relatives. These abnormalities include P50 (Cadenhead et al. 2000), P300 (McCarley et al. 1993), and N2 (Levitt et al. 1996) auditory event-related potentials; smooth pursuit eye tracking (Holzman 2000); and prepulse inhibition (Braff et al. 1999; Cadenhead et al. 1999). We focus on one psychophysiological deficit that may reflect the susceptibility to schizophrenia: the P50 sensory gating deficit.

When presented with an auditory stimulus, humans generate an electrical P50 wave response (Adler et al. 1982). If presented with two clicks 8–10 seconds apart, healthy subjects generate a diminished P50 response to the second click, termed *P50 suppression*, which is a measure of an inhibitory gating mechanism. In contrast, schizophrenic subjects fail to show a diminished P50 response to the second click, suggesting a deficit in this inhibitory gating mechanism and thus a diminished ability to filter out irrelevant sensory information (Adler et al. 1998). This deficit exists in both chronically ill schizophrenic patients and patients experiencing their first episode of schizophrenia (Yee et al. 1998), which suggests that it is not caused by the long-term effects of psychosis and is not an effect of taking antipsychotic medication. In addition, the deficit is not eliminated through treatment with typical antipsychotic medication that affects dopaminergic neurotransmission, a finding that may indicate an independent neuronal mechanism (Adler et al. 1990; Freedman et al. 1983).

P50 suppression abnormalities have been noted during the acute stages of disorders other than schizophrenia, including bipolar disorder and posttraumatic stress disorder. They have also been recorded in healthy subjects experiencing moderately severe stress. However, schizophrenia is the only disorder in which these abnormalities do not disappear during hospitalization (Adler et al. 1999; Baker et al. 1987).

Nonpsychotic parents and siblings of patients with schizophrenia show similar abnormalities in P50 suppression (Waldo et al. 1994). Initial studies involving parents showed that their P50 responses were midway between the responses of schizophrenic subjects and healthy control subjects (Siegel et al. 1984). Moreover, the likelihood of having a deficit in P50 suppression increases the more closely related an individual is to someone with schizophrenia (Waldo et al. 1991, 1995). These findings have been replicated. P50 response abnormalities in relatives closely approximated the abnormalities shown in schizophrenic subjects, and both groups differed significantly from healthy subjects (Clementz et al. 1998); these findings were also replicated. It should be noted, however, that schizophrenic patients' siblings who exhibit the P50 deficit but do not have schizophrenia may be protected by other neurobiological factors (Waldo et al. 1994).

Deficits in sensory gating are eliminated temporarily by a high dose of nicotine. Adler et al. (1993) demonstrated that schizophrenic patients who had diminished P50 gating before their first cigarette of the day had normal P50 gating after smoking approximately three cigarettes in a row. This effect lasted no more than 30 minutes after smoking. A similar transient effect was observed in schizophrenic patients' first-degree relatives who also had abnormalities in P50 suppression (Adler et al. 1992). The fact that high doses of nicotine correct abnormalities in sensory gating suggests that low-affinity nicotinic receptors are involved in sensory gating deficits (Adler et al. 1998).

Prospects and Challenges

As we have discussed in this chapter, two aspects of diagnostic criteria for schizophrenia should perhaps be reconsidered: the criteria's emphasis on psychosis, and their reliance on signs and symptoms unrelated to the disorder's etiology and pathophysiology. Changing these two aspects of schizophrenia criteria will be a radical departure from tradition and will therefore require a strong empirical foundation. The lack, until now, of such a foundation has prevented the inclusion in DSM of measures such as biological or neuropsychological abnormalities. Focusing efforts in this area will likely lead to incremental advances in the use of neurobiological diagnostic criteria.

A variety of genetic and neurobiological abnormalities may reflect the etiology (and presence) of schizophrenic illness more accurately than may clinical symptoms alone. But where should one start? The concept of schizotaxia may be especially useful in this regard. Schizotaxia is an evolving concept, not a disorder with set criteria. Tsuang et al. (1999b) recently operationalized schizotaxia criteria based on the combination of negative symptoms and neuropsychological deficits, which are two of the most robust findings in first-degree relatives of patients with schizophrenia. Nevertheless, the following criteria are tentative.

For inclusion in the schizotaxic group, subjects had to be first-degree relatives of patients with schizophrenia, speak English as a first language, have estimated IQ scores of at least 70, be between 19 and 50 years old (the age range was partly related to administration of a treatment), and give informed consent to participate. Exclusion criteria were designed to minimize the influence of comorbid neurological, psychiatric, or other medical conditions that could mimic symptoms of schizotaxia (e.g., head injuries, current substance abuse, or a history of electroconvulsive treatments). Individuals with any history of psychosis were excluded. The clinical criteria for schizotaxia involved moderate or higher levels of negative symptoms (defined as six scores of 3 or higher on the Scale for the Assessment of Negative Symptoms), and the neuropsychological criteria included moderate or greater deficits (defined as two standard deviations below normal in one cognitive domain and at least one standard deviation below normal in a second cognitive domain) in attention, long-term verbal memory, and executive function, as determined by testing. Thus, the subject's level of clinical symptoms was significant. Interestingly, none of the four cases initially reported on met criteria for any other disorder in the schizophrenia spectrum, including schizotypal personality disorder.

We hypothesized that if schizotaxia in these subjects were biologically related to schizophrenia, their schizotaxic deficits would respond to risperidone, a medication that improves negative symptoms and neuropsychological dysfunction in schizophrenic patients (see, for example, Green et al. 1997a; Rossi et al. 1997). The results were consistent with this prediction but require replication in larger, controlled studies before they can be considered as a basis for treatment. Nevertheless, the findings imply that in the future, clinical manifestations of schizotaxia may be amenable to treatment before they develop into a psychotic disorder.

This visualization of schizotaxia, if it is indeed accurate, may thus be a more specific manifestation of the predisposition to schizophrenia, compared with the DSM-IV-TR diagnosis of schizophrenia. Unlike schizophrenia, schizotaxia is not hidden by the fully advanced clinical symptoms and possible neurotoxic outcomes of psychosis that are evident in other conditions. But before schizotaxia can be incorporated into the diagnosis of schizophrenia, the predictive and concurrent validity of its criteria must be demonstrated in field trials. Given the nature of schizotaxia, researchers selecting criteria should consider dimensional as well as categorical criteria. One would assume that the biological and clinical changes that occur before psychosis begins would be covered in the criteria.

We recently performed a preliminary study of the concurrent validity of schizotaxia (Stone et al. 2001). The subjects in the study just described (Tsuang et al. 1999b) also underwent several clinical interviews, and several rating scales were used as well, in addition to tests and ratings for schizotaxia. The additional measures included the Quality of Life Scale, Social Adjustment Scale, Hopkins Symptom Checklist–90—Revised, Physical Anhedonia Scale, and Global Assessment of Functioning scale. The Social Adjustment Scale, Hopkins Symptom Checklist–90—Revised, and Physical Anhedonia Scale were all self-rated, whereas the Quality of Life Scale and Global Assessment of Functioning scale scores were determined by the investigators. As evidenced by scores on both self- and investigator-rated scales, schizotaxic subjects had consistently poorer clinical or social function. Because these findings show that schizotaxia is associated with independent measures of clinical and social function, they indicate that our specific diagnostic criteria have concurrent validity.

These results are encouraging. However, although the notion of schizotaxia is reasonable, its utility still remains something of a promissory note. Certainly, larger studies at multiple laboratories will be required to replicate our initial findings and establish the validity of the syndrome. Even if the syndrome is validated, much work will be needed to establish adequate levels of sensitivity and specificity. At present, for example, the diagnostic criteria are not very specific. There are many conditions, for example, that might produce problems in memory and attention, along with symptoms of affective constriction or asociality (e.g., attention-deficit/hyperactivity disorder and resultant emotional sequelae). This issue becomes even more evident when one considers the application of schizotaxia symptoms to a community sample. Thus far, the diagnostic criteria for schizotaxia have been applied to an "enriched" sample (i.e., relatives of patients with schizophrenia), in which the syndrome has a better likelihood of appearing than it does in the general population. Clearly, additional information will be necessary before a diagnosis of schizotaxia can be applied with confidence to conditions of individuals in the general population, such as those of unselected high school students who present with the cognitive and clinical symptoms we have described.

To some extent, the use of stringent diagnostic criteria (such as moderate or more severe symptoms in cognitive and clinical domains) in the absence of several antecedent conditions (e.g., substance abuse or known neurological conditions) reduces the likelihood of diagnostic errors (phenocopies). In the future, such an approach will not be sufficient to ensure diagnostic accuracy. It is hoped that incorporation of neurobiological measures will increase the sensitivity and specificity of the diagnosis to levels that will permit reliable and valid identification of schizotaxic individuals in both high-risk and community samples. At that point, refinements of the concept of schizotaxia will also facilitate analyses of schizotaxia's homogeneity. For instance, do schizotaxic subtypes exist among or within families, or is there a core disturbance in all affected individuals?

If more than one schizotaxic syndrome is eventually identified, other terms might be better descriptors. Nevertheless, whether *schizotaxia* or some other term is used, nosologists will need to address both the nonspecificity of psychosis and the existence of a syndrome that has a biological connection with schizophrenia. This need will become acute after interventions are developed that prevent psychosis in schizotaxic individuals (Faraone et al. 1999b).

References

Adler LE, Pachtman E, Franks R, et al: Neurophysiological evidence for a defect in neuronal mechanisms involved in sensory gating in schizophrenia. Biol Psychiatry 17:639–654, 1982

Adler LE, Gerhardt GA, Franks R, et al: Sensory physiology catecholamines in schizophrenia and mania. Psychiatry Res 31:297–309, 1990

Adler LE, Hoffer LJ, Griffith J, et al: Normalization by nicotine of deficient auditory sensory gating in the relatives of schizophrenics. Biol Psychiatry 32:607–616, 1992

Adler LE, Hoffer LJ, Wiser A, et al: Normalization of auditory physiology by cigarette smoking in schizophrenic patients. Am J Psychiatry 150:1856–1861, 1993

Adler LE, Olincy A, Waldo M, et al: Schizophrenia, sensory gating, and nicotinic receptors. Schizophr Bull 24:189–202, 1998

Adler LE, Freedman R, Ross RG, et al: Elementary phenotypes in the neurobiological and genetic study of schizophrenia. Biol Psychiatry 46:8–18, 1999

American Psychiatric Association: Diagnostic and Statistical Manual: Mental Disorders. Washington, DC, American Psychiatric Association, 1952

American Psychiatric Association: Diagnostic and Statistical Manual of Mental Disorders, 2nd Edition. Washington, DC, American Psychiatric Association, 1968

American Psychiatric Association: Diagnostic and Statistical Manual of Mental Disorders, 3rd Edition. Washington, DC, American Psychiatric Association, 1980

American Psychiatric Association: Diagnostic and Statistical Manual of Mental Disorders, 4th Edition, Text Revision. Washington, DC, American Psychiatric Association, 2000

Andreasen NC: Thought, language, and communication disorders, I: clinical assessment, definition of terms, and evaluation of their reliability. Arch Gen Psychiatry 36:1315–1321, 1979

Baker N, Adler LE, Franks RD, et al: Neurophysiological assessment of sensory gating in psychiatric inpatients: comparison between schizophrenia and other diagnoses. Biol Psychiatry 22:603–617, 1987

Bassett AS: Chromosome 5 and schizophrenia: implications for genetic linkage studies. Schizophr Bull 15:393–402, 1989

Battaglia M, Torgersen S: Schizotypal disorder: at the crossroads of genetics and nosology. Acta Psychiatr Scand 94:303–310, 1996

Battaglia M, Bernardeschi L, Franchini L, et al: A family study of schizotypal disorder. Schizophr Bull 21:33–45, 1995

Bell RC, Dudgeon P, McGorry PD, et al: The dimensionality of schizophrenia concepts in first-episode psychosis. Acta Psychiatr Scand 97:334–342, 1998

Blashfield RK: The Classification of Psychopathology: Neo-Kraepelinian and Quantitative Approaches. New York, Plenum, 1984

Braff DL, Swerdlow NR, Geyer MA: Symptom correlates of prepulse inhibition deficits in male schizophrenic patients. Am J Psychiatry 156:596–602, 1999

Brzustowicz LM, Hodgkinson KA, Chow EWC, et al: Location of a major susceptibility locus for familial schizophrenia on chromosome 1q21-q22. Science 288:678–682, 2000

Cadenhead KS, Carasso BS, Swerdlow NR, et al: Prepulse inhibition and habituation of the startle response are stable neurobiological measures in a normal male population. Biol Psychiatry 45:360–364, 1999

Cadenhead KS, Light GA, Geyer MA, et al: Sensory gating deficits assessed by the P50 event-related potential in subjects with schizotypal personality disorder. Am J Psychiatry 157:55–59, 2000

Callicott JH, Egan MF, Bertolino A, et al: Hippocampal N-acetyl aspartate in unaffected siblings of patients with schizophrenia: a possible intermediate neurobiological phenotype. Biol Psychiatry 44:941–950, 1998

Cannon TD: Abnormalities of brain structure and function in schizophrenia: implications for aetiology and pathophysiology. Ann Med 28:533–539, 1996

Cannon TD, Mednick SA, Parnas J, et al: Developmental brain abnormalities in the offspring of schizophrenic mothers, II: structural brain characteristics of schizophrenia and schizotypal personality disorder. Arch Gen Psychiatry 51:955–962, 1994a

Cannon TD, Zorrilla LE, Shtasel D, et al: Neuropsychological functioning in siblings discordant for schizophrenia and healthy volunteers. Arch Gen Psychiatry 51:651–661, 1994b

Cannon TD, Huttunen M, Standertskjold-Nordenstam CG, et al: Regional brain morphology in siblings discordant for schizophrenia: a magnetic resonance imaging study (abstract). Schizophr Res 24:140, 1997

Catts SV, McConaghy N, Ward PB, et al: Allusive thinking in parents of schizophrenics: meta-analysis. J Nerv Ment Dis 181:298–302, 1993

Chapman LJ, Chapman JP: Strategies for resolving the heterogeneity of schizophrenics and their relatives using cognitive measures. J Abnorm Psychol 98:357–366, 1989

Cichon S, Nothen MM, Rietschel M, et al: Pharmacogenetics of schizophrenia. Am J Med Genet 97:98–106, 2000

Clementz BA, Geyer MA, Braff DL: Poor P50 suppression among schizophrenia patients and their first-degree biological relatives. Am J Psychiatry 155:1691–1694, 1998

Collinge J, DeLisi LE, Boccio A, et al: Evidence for a pseudo-autosomal locus for schizophrenia using the method of affected sibling pairs. Br J Psychiatry 158:624–629, 1991

Coutts RT, Urichuk LJ: Polymorphic cytochromes P450 and drugs used in psychiatry. Cell Mol Neurobiol 19:325–354, 1999

Crow TJ: The continuum of psychosis and its genetic origins. The sixty-fifth Maudsley lecture. Br J Psychiatry 156:788–797, 1990

Crow TJ: The search for the psychosis gene. Br J Psychiatry 158:611–614, 1991

Crow TJ: From Kraepelin to Kretschmer leavened by Schneider: the transition from categories of psychosis to dimensions of variation intrinsic to *Homo sapiens*. Arch Gen Psychiatry 55:502–504, 1998a

Crow TJ: Nuclear schizophrenic symptoms as a window on the relationship between thought and speech. Br J Psychiatry 173:303–309, 1998b

DeLisi LE, Devoto M, Lofthouse R, et al: Search for linkage to schizophrenia on the X and Y chromosomes. Am J Med Genet 54:113–121, 1994

Erlenmeyer-Kimling L: Neurobehavioral deficits in offspring of schizophrenic parents: liability indicators and predictors of illness. Am J Med Genet 97:65–71, 2000

Erlenmeyer-Kimling L, Cornblatt B, Friedman D, et al: Neurological, electrophysiological, and attentional deviations in children at risk for schizophrenia, in Schizophrenia as a Brain Disease. Edited by Henn FA, Nasrallah HA. New York, Oxford University Press, 1982, pp 61–98

Faraone SV, Kremen WS, Lyons MJ, et al: Diagnostic accuracy and linkage analysis: how useful are schizophrenia spectrum phenotypes? Am J Psychiatry 152:1286–1290, 1995a

Faraone SV, Seidman LJ, Kremen WS, et al: Neuropsychological functioning among the nonpsychotic relatives of schizophrenic patients: a diagnostic efficiency analysis. J Abnorm Psychol 104:286–304, 1995b

Faraone SV, Matise T, Svrakic D, et al: Genome scan of European-American schizophrenia pedigrees: results of the NIMH Genetics Initiative and Millennium Consortium. Am J Med Genet 81:290–295, 1998

Faraone SV, Seidman LJ, Kremen WS, et al: Neuropsychological functioning among the nonpsychotic relatives of schizophrenic patients: a four-year follow-up study. J Abnorm Psychol 108:176–181, 1999a

Faraone SV, Tsuang D, Tsuang MT: Genetics of Mental Disorders: A Guide for Students, Clinicians, and Researchers. New York, Guilford, 1999b

Faraone SV, Seidman LJ, Kremen WS, et al: Neuropsychologic functioning among the nonpsychotic relatives of schizophrenic patients: the effect of genetic loading. Biol Psychiatry 48:120–126, 2000

Faraone SV, Green AI, Seidman LJ, et al: Schizotaxia: clinical implications and new directions for research. Schizophr Bull 27:1–18, 2001

Foroud T, Castellucio PF, Koller DL, et al: Genomewide scan of affected relative pairs using the NIMH Genetics Initiative bipolar affective disorder pedigrees (abstract). Am J Med Genet 81:462, 1998

Frances AJ, First MB, Widiger TA, et al: An A to Z guide to DSM-IV conundrums. J Abnorm Psychol 100:407–412, 1991

Freedman R, Adler LE, Waldo MC, et al: Neurophysiological evidence for a defect in inhibitory pathways in schizophrenia: comparison of medicated and drug-free patients. Biol Psychiatry 18:537–551, 1983

Friedman D, Squires-Wheeler E: Event-related potentials (ERPs) as indicators of risk for schizophrenia. Schizophr Bull 20:63–74, 1994

Ginns EI, Ott J, Egeland JA, et al: A genome-wide search for chromosomal loci linked to bipolar affective disorder in the Old Order Amish. Nat Genet 12:431–435, 1996

Goldberg E, Seidman LJ: Higher cortical functions in normals and in schizophrenia: a selective review, in Handbook of Schizophrenia, Vol 5. Edited by Steinhauer SR, Gruzelier JH, Zubin J. New York, Elsevier Science, 1991, pp 553–591

Goldman-Rakic PS: Prefrontal cortical dysfunction in schizophrenia: the relevance of working memory, in Psychopathology and the Brain. Edited by Carroll BJ, Barrett JE. New York, Raven, 1991

Goldman-Rakic PS: More clues to "latent" schizophrenia point to developmental origins. Am J Psychiatry 152:1701–1703, 1995

Gottesman II: Schizophrenia Genesis: The Origin of Madness. New York, Freeman, 1991

Granholm E, Asarnow RF, Marder SR: Dual task performance operating characteristics, resource limitations, and automatic processing in schizophrenia. Neuropsychology 10:11–21, 1996

Green MF, Marshall BD Jr, Wirshing WC, et al: Does risperidone improve verbal working memory in treatment resistant schizophrenia? Am J Psychiatry 154:799–804, 1997a

Green MF, Nuechterlein KH, Breitmeyer B: Backward masking performance in unaffected siblings of schizophrenic patients: evidence for a vulnerability indicator. Arch Gen Psychiatry 54:465–472, 1997b

Gunderson JG, Links PS, Reich JH: Competing models of personality disorders. J Personal Disord 5:60–68, 1991

Holzman PS: Eye movements and the search for the essence of schizophrenia. Brain Res Rev 31:350–356, 2000

Kendler KS, Karkowski LM, Walsh D: The structure of psychosis. Arch Gen Psychiatry 55:492–499, 1998

Keshavan MS, Montrose DM, Pierri JN, et al: Magnetic resonance imaging and spectroscopy in offspring at risk for schizophrenia: preliminary studies. Prog Neuropsychopharmacol Biol Psychiatry 21:1285–1295, 1997

Keverne EB: GABA-ergic neurons and the neurobiology of schizophrenia and other psychoses. Brain Res Bull 48:467–473, 1999

Knoll JL, Garver DL, Ramberg JE, et al: Heterogeneity of the psychoses: is there a neurodegenerative psychosis? Schizophr Bull 24:365–379, 1998

Kremen WS, Seidman LJ, Pepple JR, et al: Neuropsychological risk indicators for schizophrenia: a review of family studies. Schizophr Bull 20:103–119, 1994

Levitt JJ, O'Donnell BF, McCarley RW, et al: Correlations of premorbid adjustment in schizophrenia with auditory event-related potential and neuropsychological abnormalities. Am J Psychiatry 153:1347–1349, 1996

Levy DL, Holzman PS, Matthysse S, et al: Eye tracking and schizophrenia: a selective review. Schizophr Bull 20:47–62, 1994

Maier W, Lichtermann D, Minges J, et al: Continuity and discontinuity of affective disorders and schizophrenia: results of a controlled family study. Arch Gen Psychiatry 50:871–883, 1993

Maziade M, Bissonnette L, Rouillard E, et al: 6p24-22 region and major psychoses in the eastern Quebec population. Am J Med Genet 74:311–318, 1997

McCarley RW, Shenton ME, O'Donnell BF, et al: Auditory P300 abnormalities and left posterior superior temporal gyrus volume reduction in schizophrenia. Arch Gen Psychiatry 50:190–197, 1993

Meehl PE: Schizotaxia, schizotypy, schizophrenia. Am Psychol 17:827–838, 1962

Meehl PE: Schizotaxia revisited. Arch Gen Psychiatry 46:935–944, 1989

Millon T: Classification in psychopathology: rationale, alternatives, and standards. J Abnorm Psychol 100:245–261, 1991

Monti MR, Stanhellini G: Psychopathology: an edgeless razor? Compr Psychiatry 37:196–204, 1996

Motulsky AG: Drug reactions, enzymes, and biochemical genetics. JAMA 165:835–837, 1957

Nuechterlein KH, Dawson ME: Information processing and attentional functioning in the developmental course of schizophrenic disorders. Schizophr Bull 10:160–203, 1984

Parfitt E, Asherson P, Sargeant M, et al: A linkage study of the pseudoautosomal region in schizophrenia (abstract). Psychiatr Genet 2:92–93, 1991

Park S, Holzman PS, Goldman-Rakic PS: Spatial working memory deficits in the relatives of schizophrenic patients. Arch Gen Psychiatry 52:821–828, 1995

Peralta V, Cuesta MJ: Diagnostic significance of Schneider's first-rank symptoms in schizophrenia. Br J Psychiatry 174:243–248, 1998

Peralta V, Cuesta MJ, Farre C: Factor structure of symptoms in functional psychoses. Biol Psychiatry 42:806–815, 1997

Ratakonda S, Gorman JM, Yale SA, et al: Characterization of psychotic conditions: use of the domains of psychopathology model. Arch Gen Psychiatry 55:75–81, 1998

Rice JP, Goate A, Williams JT, et al: Initial genome scan of the NIMH Genetics Initiative bipolar pedigrees: chromosomes 1, 6, 8, 10, and 12. Am J Med Genet 74:247–253, 1997

Rossi A, Mancini F, Stratta P, et al: Risperidone, negative symptoms and cognitive deficit in schizophrenia: an open study. Acta Psychiatr Scand 95:40–43, 1997

Seidman LJ: The neuropsychology of schizophrenia: a neurodevelopmental and case study approach. J Neuropsychiatry Clin Neurosci 2:301–312, 1990

Seidman LJ, Cassens GP, Kremen WS, et al: Neuropsychology of schizophrenia, in Clinical Syndromes in Adult Neuropsychology: The Practitioner's Handbook. Edited by White RF. New York, Elsevier Science, 1992, pp 381–449

Seidman LJ, Breiter HC, Goldstein JM, et al: Functional MRI of attention in relatives of schizophrenic patients (abstract). Schizophr Res 24:172, 1997a

Seidman LJ, Faraone SV, Goldstein JM, et al: Reduced subcortical brain volumes in nonpsychotic siblings of schizophrenic patients: a pilot magnetic resonance imaging study. Am J Med Genet 74:507–514, 1997b

Seidman LJ, Breiter HC, Goodman JM, et al: A functional magnetic resonance imaging study of auditory vigilance with low and high information processing demands. Neuropsychology 12:505–518, 1998a

Seidman LJ, Stone WS, Jones R, et al: Comparative effects of schizophrenia and temporal lobe epilepsy on memory. J Int Neuropsychol Soc 4:342–352, 1998b

Serretti A, Macciardi F, Smeraldi E: Identification of symptomologic patterns common to major psychoses: proposal for a phenotype definition. Am J Med Genet 67:393–400, 1996

Sharma T, Lancaster E, Lee D, et al: Brain changes in schizophrenia: volumetric MRI study of families multiply affected with schizophrenia—the Maudsley Family Study 5. Br J Psychiatry 173:132–138, 1998

Sherrington R, Brynjolfsson J, Petursson H, et al: Localization of a susceptibility locus for schizophrenia on chromosome 5. Nature 336:164–167, 1988

Siegel C, Waldo M, Mizner G, et al: Deficits in sensory gating in schizophrenic patients and their relatives: evidence obtained with auditory evoked responses. Arch Gen Psychiatry 41:607–612, 1984

Stone WS, Faraone SV, Seidman LJ, et al: Concurrent validation of schizotaxia: a pilot study. Biol Psychiatry 50:434–440, 2001

Suddath RL, Christison GW, Torrey EF, et al: Anatomical abnormalities in the brains of monozygotic twins discordant for schizophrenia. N Engl J Med 322:789–794, 1990

Toomey R, Faraone SV, Seidman LJ, et al: Association of vulnerability markers in relatives of schizophrenic patients. Schizophr Res 31:89–98, 1998

Tsuang MT, Faraone SV: The case for heterogeneity in the etiology of schizophrenia. Schizophr Res 17:161–175, 1995

Tsuang MT, Stone WS, Faraone SV: Schizophrenia: a review of genetic studies. Harv Rev Psychiatry 7:185–207, 1999a

Tsuang MT, Stone WS, Seidman LJ, et al: Treatment of nonpsychotic relatives of patients with schizophrenia: four case studies. Biol Psychiatry 41:1412–1418, 1999b

Waldo MC, Carey G, Myles-Worsley M, et al: Codistribution of a sensory gating deficit and schizophrenia in multi-affected families. Psychiatry Res 39:257–268, 1991

Waldo MC, Cawthra E, Adler LE, et al: Auditory sensory gating, hippocampal volume, and catecholamine metabolism in schizophrenics and their siblings. Schizophr Res 12:93–106, 1994

Waldo M[C], Myles-Worsley M, Madison A, et al: Sensory gating deficits in parents of schizophrenics. Am J Med Genet 60:506–511, 1995

Weinberger DR: Implications of normal brain development for the pathogenesis of schizophrenia. Arch Gen Psychiatry 44:660–669, 1987

Weinberger DR: Schizophrenia as a neurodevelopmental disorder: a review of the concept, in Schizophrenia. Edited by Hirsch SR, Weinberger DR. London, Blackwood, 1994, pp 293–323

Weinberger DR: Neurodevelopmental perspectives on schizophrenia, in Psychopharmacology: The Fourth Generation of Progress. Edited by Bloom FE, Kupfer DJ. New York, Raven, 1995, pp 1171–1183

Wildenauer D[B], Hallmayer J, Albus M: A susceptibility locus for affective and schizophrenic disorder? (abstract) Psychiatr Genet 6:152, 1996

Wildenauer DB, Schwab SG, Maier W, et al: Do schizophrenia and affective disorder share susceptibility genes? Schizophr Res 39:107–111, 1999

Woods BT: Is schizophrenia a progressive neurodevelopmental disorder? toward a unitary pathogenetic mechanism. Am J Psychiatry 155:1661–1670, 1998

Wyatt RJ: Early intervention for schizophrenia: can the course of the illness be altered? Biol Psychiatry 38:1–3, 1995

Yee CM, Nuechterlein KH, Morris SE, et al: P50 suppression in recent onset schizophrenia: clinical correlates and risperidone effects. J Abnorm Psychol 107:691–698, 1998

CHAPTER 6

Subthreshold Mental Disorders

Nosological and Research Recommendations

Harold Alan Pincus, M.D., Laurie E. McQueen, M.S.S.W., Lynn Elinson, Ph.D.

D SM-III (American Psychiatric Association 1980) introduced a new paradigm for establishing diagnoses in psychiatry—one involving the use of objective, operationalized criteria with specific thresholds. Greater reliability in diagnosis was achieved, and communication improved among clinicians and among researchers regarding whether an individual had a mental disorder, or, in epidemiological terms, whether a case of mental disorder existed. The primary focus of DSM-III is on populations presenting for treatment in mental health care settings. Questions have repeatedly been raised about whether the specifically delineated disorders in DSM-III, in the later DSM editions, and in the *International Statistical Classification of Diseases and Related Health Problems*, 10th Revision (ICD-10; World Health Organization 1992) capture the full spectrum of psychopathology in the general population and in primary care settings, as well as in the mental health care setting (deGruy and Pincus 1996).

In recognition of the limitations in their coverage, DSM and ICD-10 include "not otherwise specified" (NOS) categories, into which atypical conditions or conditions not meeting full criteria for a specific mental dis-

Portions of this chapter are reprinted with permission from Pincus HA, Davis WW, McQueen LE: "'Subthreshold' Mental Disorders: A Review and Synthesis of Studies on Minor Depression and Other 'Brand Names.'" *British Journal of Psychiatry* 174:288–296, 1999. Used with permission.

order are placed. Nonetheless, there have been continual calls for the addition of other new "disorders." When DSM-IV (American Psychiatric Association 1994) was being constructed, more than 150 new disorders were proposed, with varying levels of evidence supporting their addition to the classification (Pincus et al. 1992).

Subthreshold forms of depression are particularly important because of their prevalence, clinical significance, and cost. Studies have demonstrated that depressive symptoms in various combinations, including subthreshold conditions, are present in as much as 24% of the population (Horwarth et al. 1992). Not only are the numbers of individuals with subthreshold depressive syndromes quite large, but the degree of morbidity and functional impairment is extensive. Wells et al. (1989) found that although the degree of impairment associated with subthreshold depressive symptoms is somewhat less than that associated with major depressive disorder, it is comparable to the level of impairment associated with other medical conditions. In addition, individuals whose symptoms do not meet full criteria for major depressive disorder manifest high rates of service utilization and medical care costs (Johnson et al. 1992). Finally, the characterization of minor forms of depression provides an opportunity to identify individuals potentially at risk for more severe forms of the disorder and to develop interventions that might prevent more extensive morbidity.

Minor forms of depression have not been a major focus within the mental health care community, because most individuals with these conditions present to primary care providers, or seek no treatment, rather than see mental health care professionals. In fact, a continuing problem in the relationship between primary care providers and mental health care providers is that each group is often looking at different parts of the "elephant" of mental morbidity. Primary care physicians see more subthreshold conditions, whereas mental health care professionals see the more severe end of the spectrum. Some attempts to break down these barriers have been made, as evidenced by books such as *Diagnostic and Statistical Manual of Mental Disorders, Fourth Edition, Primary Care Version* (DSM-IV-PC; American Psychiatric Association 1995) and *Diagnostic and Management Guidelines for Mental Disorders in Primary Care: ICD-10 Chapter V Primary Care Version* (World Health Organization 1996). However, these two works are based on DSM-IV and the ICD-10 Diagnostic Criteria for Research (DCR), respectively, and do not include new nosological approaches for dealing with subthreshold conditions. An increased focus in this area may help to better link the primary care and mental health care communities in terms of research and clinical care.

In this chapter, we discuss the complicating factors and issues that surround the identification of subthreshold mental conditions. We use depression as a paradigm for other conditions that have subthreshold features. We begin the chapter by defining subthreshold conditions and describing their characterizations in both DSM-IV-TR (American Psychiatric Association 2000) (the latest DSM) and ICD-10. We then discuss a systematic review of the literature on subthreshold conditions for depression (Pincus et al. 1999), update this review by considering more recent publications, and present a clinical perspective on the heterogeneity of subthreshold conditions. Finally, we raise a number of nosological considerations regarding diagnostic classification of subthreshold conditions, and with these considerations in mind, we make recommendations for improving research.

Definitions

Subthreshold conditions are included in DSM-IV-TR and ICD-10, although they are not always specifically delineated. For example, subthreshold depressive conditions are subsumed under the category of depression NOS. The definition of *mental disorder* in DSM-IV-TR, however, states that there must be clinically significant impairment or distress. To highlight the importance of considering this issue, criteria sets for many disorders include a "clinical significance" criterion, usually worded "causes clinically significant distress or impairment in social, occupational, or other important areas of functioning." This criterion helps establish a threshold for the diagnosis of a disorder in situations in which the symptomatic presentation by itself (particularly in its milder forms) is not pathological and may be encountered in individuals for whom a diagnosis of mental disorder would be inappropriate (Frances 1998). The "solution" of applying this criterion is not without problems (see Chapter 2 in this volume, "Clarifying the Distinction Between Disorder and Nondisorder"; Spitzer and Wakefield 1999).

For the purposes of this discussion, subthreshold conditions are conditions that do not meet the full symptomatic or duration criteria for a specific disorder but do meet the DSM-IV-TR clinical significance criterion (i.e., cause clinically significant distress or impairment). Subthreshold conditions, as defined here, would be placed within the corresponding NOS category in DSM-IV-TR. For example, Appendix B in DSM-IV-TR ("Criteria Sets and Axes Provided for Further Study") includes a number of criteria sets for subthreshold depressive conditions (e.g., minor depressive disorder and recurrent brief depressive disorder) that would be categorized under depressive disorder NOS.

Minor depressive disorder is defined in DSM-IV-TR as the presence of at least two, but fewer than five, depressive symptoms (one symptom must be either depressed mood or loss of interest) during the same 2-week period, with no history of major depressive episode or dysthymic disorder. *Recurrent brief depressive disorder* is defined as the presence of depressive episodes (i.e., five of the nine possible symptoms of major depressive episode) for less than 2 weeks, with the episodes occurring at least once a month for 12 consecutive months. The primary differences between these two definitions concern the number of symptoms needed for a diagnosis and the duration of those symptoms.

If the subthreshold symptoms occur as a maladaptive reaction to a stressful event, a diagnosis of adjustment disorder with depressed mood is made (unless the symptoms occur in the context of bereavement, in which case a V code is applied).

The subthreshold conditions just discussed are distinguished from what might be termed *subclinical conditions*, in which symptoms of a mental disorder may occur but do not cause clinically significant distress or impairment. In contrast to subthreshold conditions, subclinical conditions are not placed in NOS categories but instead are categorized as "Other Conditions That May Be a Focus of Clinical Attention" (which include V-code diagnoses) or simply listed using symptom codes (e.g., Sadness).

Adding to this diagnostic confusion are differences between DSM-IV-TR and ICD-10 DCR. In ICD-10 DCR, depressive episodes are defined by symptom thresholds and are subtyped "mild," "moderate," or "severe" according to the number of symptoms (i.e., 4 of 10 symptoms for mild, 6 of 10 for moderate, and 8 of 10 for severe). Also, the symptoms need not cause clinically significant distress or impairment. This lower symptom threshold for mild depressive disorder (i.e., 4 of 10 symptoms vs. 5 of 9 symptoms for DSM-IV-TR major depressive disorder of any severity) may blur the boundary between major depressive disorder and a subthreshold condition as defined in DSM-IV-TR (e.g., the NOS variant of minor depression in Appendix B). There is no symptom threshold or clinical significance criterion in ICD-10 DCR for the "unspecified depression" categories (the rough equivalent of NOS categories in DSM-IV-TR). ICD-10 does include both brief recurrent depression and mixed anxiety depression, but no criteria are specified for the latter.

A Systematic Review

To illustrate the confusion and complexity regarding subthreshold conditions, Pincus et al. (1999) recently published a systematic review of subthreshold depression categories. Using the index terms *diagnosis, subthreshold mental disorders, minor depression, mixed anxiety depression, recurrent brief depression,* or *recurrent brief depressive disorder,* they conducted a *MEDLINE* search for articles published between January 1991 and December 1995. Relevant references from these reports were also considered. Reports of studies of bereavement, adjustment disorder, depressive personality disorder, and dysthymic disorder were not included in the review unless the studies also examined minor depression or brief recurrent depression.

This selection process yielded 36 reports of studies that considered the characteristics and defining features of individuals with a subthreshold or "minor" depressive condition. The authors abstracted from each article the definition of *subthreshold condition* in terms of 1) the criteria used to describe the condition, 2) the minimum duration of symptoms, 3) whether impairment was a criterion, and 4) what other conditions or stressors that might potentially explain the symptoms were ruled out. The number and source of subjects, comparison groups, the study design, and reliability assessment were also considered. Finally, the authors examined the studies' findings on the prevalence, course, and impairment associated with the conditions studied.

Symptom Sets and Thresholds

The authors found that subthreshold depressive conditions have many definitions and names. In several instances, different symptom sets were given the same name; conversely, different names were sometimes given to the same symptom set. For example, *minor depression* (or *minor depressive disorder, minor depression with mood disturbance, or minor depression without mood disturbance*—terms that were also used) was defined nine ways, with three sets of studies sharing definitions. Five definitions were provided for *subthreshold depression* (or *subthreshold depressive disorder, subsyndromal depression, or subsyndromal symptomatic depression*). There were three definitions of *depressive symptoms* (or *subthreshold depressive symptoms* or *depression symptoms only*), with two studies sharing one definition. *Mixed anxiety depression* was defined two ways, with two studies sharing a definition. Two definitions were used in two articles in which depression NOS was described. Two symptom lists were used for recurrent brief depression (also called *brief depression, subthreshold recurrent brief depression,* and *recurrent brief depression—seasonal*). Angst's criteria (Angst et al. 1990) were used in eight studies, and ICD-10 DCR were used in one study.

The minimum number of symptoms required for a diagnosis of one of the subthreshold conditions ranged from one to six, although the most common minimum was two (five for recurrent brief depression). In more than half the studies, depressed mood, and often anhedonia, were required for a diagnosis. In some studies, screening questionnaires were used to determine the presence of a subthreshold condition. The Beck Depression Inventory, Center for Epidemiologic Studies Depression Scale, Hamilton

Rating Scale for Depression, Hamilton Anxiety Scale, and Inventory to Diagnose Depression were used.

Duration

In 13 articles, the authors did not report a required duration of symptoms. Of the articles in which a duration criterion was reported, 11 included a requirement of 2 weeks of symptoms. These 11 articles included different symptom sets and varying names. In one study, 10 days of symptoms were required; in another study, symptoms had to be present for a month.

In seven studies of brief recurrent depression, a duration of symptoms of less than 2 weeks was noted, but symptom sets and requirements for recurrence varied. In one of these studies, a definition of *recurrent brief depression* ("frequent") was used that allowed for recurrence of symptoms "frequently but not every month in the past year." In one study, episodes of less than 2 weeks' duration, occurring monthly throughout the fall and winter, were required if the symptom set was to be considered recurrent brief depression. In an additional study, episodes (defined as "recurrent brief depression") occurred monthly over a year's time but were of less than a week's duration.

Impairment

In 25 of the 36 studies surveyed, an impairment criterion was not included (or was not reported to be included) in the definition of the featured subthreshold condition. In the remaining 11 studies, at least one of the following was required: treatment-seeking behavior; clinically significant distress; psychosocial impairment; impairment in occupational, social, or general functioning; or subjective distress as measured by the General Health Questionnaire.

Exclusions

The authors also considered which and how often other diagnoses were ruled out before a diagnosis of a subthreshold depressive condition could be made. Only two studies considered the potential role of a stressor in the depressive symptoms seen, and these studies specifically focused on cancer patients and patients with coronary heart disease.

Other Study Characteristics

The settings in which data were collected included primary care settings, mental health care settings, inpatient settings, and mixed settings (e.g., primary care settings with an on-site mental health care provider). Several studies were community-based epidemiological studies, with sample sizes ranging from 25 to 18,571 individuals. Few studies (other than treatment studies) followed patients longitudinally, and little information was available on the course of their conditions. In only two articles was a statistic for the reliability of diagnostic criteria reported. Prevalence rates for different symptoms (in the case of articles with a prevalence statistic) were highly variable across the various definitions and settings, ranging from 0.8% to 52.6%. Twenty-one of 30 articles did not provide information on impairment associated with these conditions.

Conclusions From the Literature Review

The overall conclusion drawn from this review is that there is much confusion and complexity in the nosological characterization of subthreshold depressive conditions. There are a myriad of definitions for subthreshold conditions, with varying durations and symptom thresholds; and prevalence rates vary widely, according to the setting and populations studied. Moreover, the existing studies are methodologically weak. For example, few articles on these studies included information on the course of the conditions or on the level of impairment, and rarely was the context of the symptoms considered.

Because this review focused on articles published between 1991 and 1995, we undertook the examination of reports of studies of minor or subthreshold depression that were published in English-language journals after 1995. After eliminating review articles and articles that were reanalyses of data collected and categorized before 1996, we had a total of 52 reports. In these studies, minor depression was diagnosed using DSM-III or DSM-III-R (American Psychiatric Association 1987) criteria (23 studies), DSM-IV criteria (20 studies), DSM-III and DSM-IV criteria (2 studies), Research Diagnostic Criteria (RDC) (5 studies), and other categorizing schemata (2 studies).

Of the reports of studies in which DSM-IV criteria were used, nine included the number of symptoms needed to meet a diagnosis of minor depression (namely, one to three symptoms, two to four symptoms, two or more symptoms, and three to four symptoms). Duration criteria were specified in three articles, and the authors of one report specifically indicated a clinical significance threshold, such as functional impairment. In none of these articles was it stated that a longitudinal perspective (e.g., assessment of previous episodes of major depression) was used. As a result, it was unclear whether subjects who had prior episodes of major depression were categorized as having major depression in partial remission rather than minor depression.

Although this new review indicates a certain amount of compliance with standardized diagnostic criteria for minor depression subsequent to the publication of DSM-IV, such compliance appears to be related primarily to symptom counts. Duration of symptoms as a criterion is used less often, and a clinical significance threshold and a longitudinal approach are used even less. In this more recent literature review, there may actually have been a bias toward finding an increased use of DSM-IV and DSM-IV-TR criteria for minor depression, because reports of studies without rigorous criteria for identifying subthreshold or minor depression may not have been published. In addition, this exercise may indicate the extent to which precise diagnostic criteria are used in research, but it does not provide information on the manner in which community physicians diagnose minor depression.

Clinical Perspectives on the Heterogeneity of Subthreshold Conditions

In most research studies, investigators evaluate patients using some type of standardized assessment instrument. However, most of these studies are imprecise in terms of diagnostic categorization. Although standardization obviously has important advantages, failure to systematically consider specific nosological issues limits the extension of research findings across studies and the application of these findings to clinical practice. For example, given the variations in patient presentation, a clinician could reasonably question the assessment of subthreshold depression in studies, as follows:

- Was there sufficient inquiry into whether all the symptoms of major depressive disorder were assessed in an appropriate way?
- Was a longitudinal perspective built into the assessment that would reflect whether a major depressive episode had occurred earlier and whether there was partial remission? Might some patients with a diagnosis of subthreshold depressive disorder actually have major depression in partial remission?
- Has the individual had a recurrent form of major depression, and is he or she currently experiencing a partial relapse?
- Might a fluctuation in the occurrence of symptoms exist but not have been fully recalled by the patient in the presence of the assessor?
- Were other disorders with similar symptoms (e.g., depressive personality disorder, dysthymic disorder, bereavement, or adjustment disorder) considered and ruled out? Was the context of these symptoms fully considered? For example, did symptoms occur in connection with another

mental disorder or severe social, economic, or occupational problems, or in relation to a significant general medical condition?

- Does the depression-related term used in the study fully characterize the syndrome studied? For example, were these subthreshold depressive symptoms occurring alongside other types of symptoms (e.g., anxiety symptoms or somatization symptoms)? Would other cultures refer to these symptoms in a different way (e.g., using the term *neurasthenia* to refer to fatigue and malaise)?
- Was any attempt made to characterize the significance and pervasiveness of depressive symptoms with regard to the symptoms' effects on the patients' lives (e.g., do the symptoms cause clinically significant impairment)?
- To what extent might these symptoms be normal mood fluctuations, given a broader understanding of the patient's experience?

Clearly, lack of attention to issues such as these has made interpretation of studies of subthreshold depression problematic and imprecise. Much work still needs to be done to clarify and better standardize the diagnosis and categorization of subthreshold depression. Because it has become more apparent during the last several years that there are significant differences in treatment response between major and subthreshold forms of depression, the need to refine these complexities is even more pressing.

Future Nosological Considerations

Several specific nosological issues pertaining to subthreshold depression need to be addressed, and some changes might be considered for future diagnostic classifications. These issues are presented here and are intended to stimulate further thinking and research so that revisions of diagnostic classifications can be made in the future.

Adjustment Disorder

According to DSM-IV-TR, "the essential feature of an Adjustment Disorder is a psychological response to an identifiable stressor or stressors that results in the development of clinically significant emotional or behavioral symptoms" (American Psychiatric Association 2000, p. 679). Applying the criteria for adjustment disorder requires establishing linkage among a stressful event, the presence of subthreshold symptoms, and a maladaptive response. Such an assessment—and, thus, distinguishing adjustment disorder with, for example, depressive mood from minor depressive disorder—is inherently subjective and unreliable. More importantly, it is assumed in the current nosology that adjustment disorder and minor depression are two separate entities.

One approach to these problems would be to eliminate the category of adjustment disorder altogether and maintain a category of subthreshold conditions within each of the major phenomenological groupings of DSM-IV-TR and ICD-10 DCR (e.g., anxiety, depressive, cognitive, and somatoform disorders). Subtyping in relationship to the presence of a stressor would then be permitted. This approach is similar to the DSM-IV-TR approach to brief psychotic disorder. The proposed approach would be noncommittal about whether adjustment disorder and each phenomenological group are distinct. In other words, the approach keeps all the data available without forcing a decision. Although this approach would add some degree of complexity, it would allow data to be more reliably and systematically collected to help resolve the issue.

Comorbidity

Comorbidity of DSM disorders is common and may reflect a limitation in the classification system's ability to portray syndromal complexity. The extent of comorbidity is greater among subthreshold conditions, in that distinctions among diagnostic groups diminish at lower severities (see, for example, Moras et al. 1996). Thus, many individuals have combinations of somatoform, anxiety, depressive, and/or dissociative symptoms. There are several approaches that might be applied specifically to subthreshold conditions occurring with other conditions.

Using combination categories such as mixed anxiety and depressive disorder or mixed somatoform and depressive disorder is a simple approach that would be particularly useful in primary care settings. However, there is not much of a tradition of using combination categories in the United States. More complex, though potentially more valid, approaches are possible (such as the use of dimensional models, in which the classification of clinical presentations is based on quantifying attributes), but these approaches represent an even greater break with the past. Alternatively, the number of recognized subthreshold categories in DSM-IV-TR could be expanded, and a nonhierarchical listing of multiple conditions could be permitted. With this alternative, the traditional approach would be retained, but patients could have a greatly expanded number of diagnoses. At the subthreshold level, there are limited data for choosing among these.

Subthreshold Diagnoses in the Context of General Medical Conditions

General medical conditions (such as coronary artery disease [Ariyo et al. 2000]) may result from depression. Conversely, many (if not all) significant general medical conditions cause some degree of depressive symptomatology, either directly (e.g., a patient with congestive heart failure may have sleep problems because of dyspnea) or indirectly (e.g., a diabetic individual whose foot has been amputated may be disheartened by his or her loss of function). As a result, a number of diagnostic issues have been identified (von Ammon Cavanaugh 1995). These issues have been explored with regard to major depressive disorder (and other conditions), and solutions have been unsatisfying. For example, investigators have used "inclusive," "exclusive," and "substitutive" approaches. In the inclusive approach, all symptoms—regardless of their presumed etiology—are included in an assessment of psychiatric conditions. In the exclusive approach, symptoms caused by medical problems are excluded. In the substitutive approach, psychological symptoms are substituted for physical symptoms that may be somatic. The inclusive approach is applied to major depression in DSM-IV-TR.

Subthreshold Diagnoses in the Context of Suprathreshold Mental Disorders

Many individuals with Axis I or II conditions also manifest symptoms of another Axis I condition at a subthreshold level (e.g., patients with borderline personality disorder or social phobia [social anxiety disorder] might have two to three depressive symptoms). Should there be a convention for listing these subthreshold conditions? Would the advantages of such an approach outweigh the additional burden to the clinician of making such diagnoses?

Clinical Significance

The current definition of *mental disorder* requires that there be clinically significant distress or impairment. Changing the conjunction *or* to *and*, as well as requiring some objective impairment in major role functioning, might be a way of ensuring that a diagnosis is applied only when there is evidence of clinical significance.

For example, one could specify that for subthreshold syndromes to be considered disorders, some obvious (and, it is to be hoped, systematic and reliable) evidence of impairment or dysfunction must be present. Such an approach would prevent labeling as mentally ill large groups of individuals who might not see themselves as having a mental disorder (and who might neither seek treatment nor be impaired). (This "false-positives" problem is discussed in Chapter 2 in this volume, "Clarifying the Distinction Between Disorder and Nondisorder.")

Developing an objective, reliable, and valid definition of *impairment* is a major challenge in itself. Moreover, if a new class of subthreshold disorders is explicitly added to the official nomenclature, the apparent prevalence of mental disorders would likely increase without a great deal of evidence regarding the validity of these "newly discovered" conditions.

Longitudinality

Too often, in both research and clinical situations, individuals are assessed with a single instrument at one point in time. The problem with this approach is that some conditions have fluctuating symptoms and are recurrent. A onetime assessment does not indicate where the patient is in terms of the condition's longitudinal course. One way to solve this problem is to require a longitudinal or course perspective. Moving away from cross-sectional symptom reports (e.g., diagnosing multiple sclerosis with two points in time and space) might improve diagnostic validity. However, this approach might be at the expense of reliability, given the limitations of retrospective accounts.

Categorization of Symptoms

In principle, clinicians could apply the current *International Classification of Diseases*, 9th Revision (ICD-9-CM; World Health Organization 1978) 780 symptom codes (or R codes in ICD-10) to record their "diagnosis" for many subthreshold conditions. Using symptom codes discourages premature closure on a diagnosis and encourages a clinical strategy of watchful waiting, complementary to the longitudinal perspective noted in the preceding paragraph. Use of these codes might result in a more extensive data collection process, capturing the patterning of symptoms. On the other hand, if clinicians recorded all the symptoms of subthreshold conditions, the classification scheme would be too cumbersome. In addition, most reimbursement systems do not permit such categorization on an official basis.

Simplification

Unfortunately, many of the suggestions presented here would make the system of disorder identification more complex rather than simpler. Additional complexity would make the process much more difficult for primary care providers, who face limitations in both time and knowledge, given the myriad of preventive and subspecialty expectations. For the diagnostic system to be used, it may be necessary to develop separate approaches for research and clinical care (and primary care as well). Of course, such an approach could lead to increasing separation of these communities and a lack of communication.

The Term *Subthreshold*

The terms *subthreshold condition* and *minor depression* carry implications of triviality and lack of importance. Other terms, such as *limited depression, sub-depression,* and *boundary depression,* do not appear to be much better. Another approach, similar to that taken by the World Health Organization (1997), would be to expand the concept of dysthymia beyond that of chronic mild depression, to incorporate acute, subchronic, and chronic forms.

Recommendations for Future Research

The next generation of studies of minor depression must be more methodologically and intellectually rigorous if these clinical issues are to be better addressed, and greater consideration must be given to the place of these subthreshold conditions in the context of broader clinical and nosological issues. The use of objective criteria and new assessment instruments allows for increased precision in psychiatric assessment. However, breaking syndromes into more elemental subsets of criteria may accelerate the trend toward viewing as medical and pathological those conditions that lie within the normal spectrum. Furthermore, the profusion of approaches to categorizing various subthreshold conditions—approaches often only slightly different from one another—adds a perhaps unnecessary complexity to the system. These concerns are multiplied as the issues illustrated in terms of minor depression are replicated for disorders such as anxiety disorders, cognitive disorders, and somatoform disorders. Thus, this rush to identify a named syndrome may undercut the ability to assess individual patients holistically. Finally, the varying approaches to defining and studying these conditions may inhibit communication between psychiatrists and primary care providers. Most studies are conducted by psychiatry-based investigators or primary care–based investigators. Very few involve interdisciplinary collaboration or the collection of samples from multiple settings.

Therefore, we recommend the following:

• The rush to create diagnoses for subthreshold conditions should be halted. Investigators should examine these syndromes from a broad perspective, not with the intent of promoting a single specific conceptualization. At a minimum, data collection should allow the conceptual and empirical "mapping" of specific currently defined syndromes onto other ways of defining these conditions, as well as assessment of the broader context (e.g., assessment of general medical conditions, longitudinality, or stressors).

- When considering subthreshold conditions, investigators should systematically assess an array of key variables, including symptom thresholds; duration of symptoms; psychosocial impairment; impairment in occupational or social functioning; course; family history; and comorbidity with other mental disorders and general medical conditions.

- Longitudinal designs must be promoted. Little is known about the natural history and course of subthreshold conditions. Are they self-limited risk factors for more severe conditions, or do they have a stable course? Furthermore, virtually nothing is known about the effects of treatment, both psychosocial and psychopharmacological. Clinical, epidemiological, longitudinal, natural history, and treatment studies (with placebo control subjects and perhaps untreated control subjects or the use of watchful waiting) should adhere to the same principles for comprehensive, systematic assessment and descriptions noted here.

Primary Care and Psychiatry

Further research is especially needed to help illuminate the boundary between primary care and psychiatry. Although primary care physicians and mental health clinicians may agree about the presence or absence of a mental health diagnosis in most instances, there are also clear discrepancies, with false negatives and false positives from both perspectives. A series of studies indicate that primary care physicians often fail to recognize major depression and other conditions identified by specialists (Kirmayer et al. 1993; Regier et al. 1993). There remains some dispute about whether this reflects a failure to recognize conditions, whether this indicates a failure of the patient to acknowledge symptoms (Klinkman 1997), or whether these conditions are recognized but simply not noted in the chart (Rost et al. 1994).

In addition, there are clearly a number of mental disorders, conditions, and psychosocial factors that primary care physicians think are very important but that are not well articulated in the psychiatric nosology and are often not a major consideration of mental health specialists. These need to be more systematically explored. Investigators also need to consider the multiaxial system (i.e., the role of Axis IV psychosocial stressors), as well as the interaction of psychiatric symptoms with Axis III general medical syndromes. Finally, further nosological and scientific development should involve multidisciplinary groups that incorporate primary care, psychiatry, and other behavioral sciences.

Conclusion

There is much evidence to support the notion that subthreshold conditions are important public health problems. However, a great deal more research is needed to clarify diagnostic boundaries across the range of subthreshold and suprathreshold conditions and normality. It is to be hoped that by the time the next revisions of DSM-IV-TR and ICD-10 DCR classifications are initiated, a broader, more systematic, and well-documented empirical base will be available for making nosological decisions.

References

American Psychiatric Association: Diagnostic and Statistical Manual of Mental Disorders, 3rd Edition. Washington, DC, American Psychiatric Association, 1980

American Psychiatric Association: Diagnostic and Statistical Manual of Mental Disorders, 3rd Edition, Revised. Washington, DC, American Psychiatric Association, 1987

American Psychiatric Association: Diagnostic and Statistical Manual of Mental Disorders, 4th Edition. Washington, DC, American Psychiatric Association, 1994

American Psychiatric Association: Diagnostic and Statistical Manual of Mental Disorders, Fourth Edition, Primary Care Version. Washington, DC, American Psychiatric Association, 1995

American Psychiatric Association: Diagnostic and Statistical Manual of Mental Disorders, 4th Edition, Text Revision. Washington, DC, American Psychiatric Association, 2000

Angst J, Merikangas K, Scheiddeger P, et al: Recurrent brief depression: a new subtype of affective disorder. J Affect Disord 19:87–98, 1990

Ariyo AA, Haan M, Tangen CM, et al: Depressive symptoms and risks of coronary artery disease mortality in elderly Americans. Cardiovascular Health Study Collaborative Research Group. Circulation 102:1773–1779, 2000

deGruy FV 3rd, Pincus H: The DSM-IV-PC: a manual for diagnosing mental disorders in the primary care setting. J Am Board Fam Pract 9:274–281, 1996

Frances A: Problems in defining clinical significance in epidemiological studies (comment). Arch Gen Psychiatry 55:119, 1998

Horwarth E, Johnson J, Klerman GL, et al: Depressive symptoms as relative and attributable risk factors for first-onset major depression. Arch Gen Psychiatry 49:817–823, 1992

Johnson J, Weissman MM, Klerman GL: Service utilization and social morbidity associated with depressive symptoms in the community. JAMA 267:1478–1483, 1992

Kirmayer LJ, Robbins JM, Dworkind M, et al: Somatization and the recognition of depression and anxiety in primary care. Am J Psychiatry 150:734–741, 1993

Klinkman MS: Competing demands in psychosocial care: a model for the identification and treatment of depressive disorders in primary care. Gen Hosp Psychiatry 19:98–111, 1997

Moras K, Clark LA, Katon W, et al: Mixed anxiety-depression, in DSM-IV Sourcebook, Vol 2. Edited by Widiger TA, Frances AJ, Pincus HA, et al. Washington, DC, American Psychiatric Association, 1996, pp 623–643

Pincus HA, Frances A, Davis WW, et al: DSM-IV and new diagnostic categories: holding the line on proliferation. Am J Psychiatry 149:112–117, 1992

Pincus HA, Davis WW, McQueen LE: "Subthreshold" mental disorders: a review and synthesis of studies on minor depression and other "brand names." Br J Psychiatry 174:288–296, 1999

Regier DA, Narrow WE, Rae DS, et al: The de facto US mental health and addictive disorders service system: Epidemiologic Catchment Area prospective 1-year prevalence rates of disorders and services. Arch Gen Psychiatry 50:85–94, 1993

Rost K, Smith R, Matthews DB, et al: The deliberate misdiagnosis of major depression. Arch Fam Med 3:333–337, 1994

Spitzer RL, Wakefield JC: DSM-IV diagnostic criterion for clinical significance: does it help solve the false positives problem? Am J Psychiatry 156:1856–1864, 1999

von Ammon Cavanaugh S: Depression in the medically ill: critical issues in diagnostic assessment. Psychosomatics 36:48–49, 1995

Wells KB, Stewart A, Hays RD, et al: The functioning and well-being of depressed patients: results from the Medical Outcomes Study. JAMA 262:914–919, 1989

World Health Organization: International Classification of Diseases, 9th Revision, Clinical Modification. Ann Arbor, MI, Commission on Professional and Hospital Activities, 1978

World Health Organization: International Statistical Classification of Diseases and Related Health Problems, 10th Revision. Geneva, World Health Organization, 1992

World Health Organization: Diagnostic and Management Guidelines for Mental Disorders in Primary Care: ICD-10 Chapter V Primary Care Version. Seattle, WA, Hogrefe & Huber Publishers, 1996 (Description and codes available at : http://www.who.int/msa/mnh/ems/icd10/icd10.htm#codes. Accessed August 5, 2002)

World Health Organization: Classification of Dysthymia and Related Conditions in Neurological Diseases: Recommendations for the Clinical Descriptions and Criteria for Research—Version for Field Trials. Geneva, Division of Mental Health and Prevention of Substance Abuse, World Health Organization, 1997

CHAPTER 7

Multiaxial Assessment in the Twenty-First Century

Alan M. Gruenberg, M.D., Reed D. Goldstein, Ph.D.

A multiaxial system of evaluation was officially introduced in psychiatry with the publication of DSM-III (American Psychiatric Association 1980). This system encouraged the evaluation of patients from a variety of clinical and phenomenological perspectives. The approach included identifying specific clinical psychiatric syndromes on Axis I, characterizing personality attributes on Axis II, delineating nonpsychiatric medical conditions on Axis III, coding psychosocial stressors on Axis IV, and estimating psychosocial functioning on Axis V. The multiaxial format was introduced to encourage clinicians to provide an "evaluation to ensure that certain information that may be of value in planning treatment and predicting outcome for each individual is recorded on each of five axes" (p. 8).

Before the development of DSM-IV (American Psychiatric Association 1994), the Multiaxial Issues Work Group was formed (Williams 1997). The group evaluated the current multiaxial system of evaluation, addressed its continued utility, and considered reasons for its relative lack of use in clinical settings. The work group concluded that 1) the system did not facilitate comprehensive evaluation, 2) there was no consistent form for clinicians or institutions to code all five axes, 3) clinicians did not receive sufficient training to make ratings on all five axes (especially Axes III and IV), and 4) the coding of all axes in clinical settings was infrequent (Williams 1997).

DSM-IV reflected other deliberations of the Multiaxial Issues Work Group. Pervasive developmental disorders in childhood, which were listed on Axis II in DSM-III-R (American Psychiatric Association 1987), were listed on Axis I in DSM-IV. The work group continued to support a separate axis for personality disorders on Axis II. It recognized that certain Axis II personality disorders are genetically linked to Axis I conditions and that certain Axis II personality disorders have fundamental neurobiological components. However, the group supported maintaining a separate axis to facilitate empirical research on personality disorders. No changes for coding Axis III were made in DSM-IV, but the work group challenged clinicians to delineate all relevant nonpsychiatric medical conditions. The most radical change in the DSM-IV multiaxial system related to Axis IV. The DSM-III-R rating of severity of stressors was replaced by a checklist for identifying current stressors, such as interpersonal losses, problems with housing, legal problems, and employment difficulties. The reasons for this change included the unreliability of rating severity of stressors, the inconsistent use of these ratings across settings and among clinicians, and the questionable utility of these ratings in predicting outcome. The clinician was now instructed to list all significant psychosocial stressors that may be relevant to the current clinical condition. Finally, with regard to Axis V, the work group endorsed the continued use of the Global Assessment of Functioning (GAF) scale. In addition, DSM-IV included a multiaxial report form, to be used in clinical or administrative settings.

DSM-IV-TR (American Psychiatric Association 2000) was published in 2000. The text includes a stepwise approach for determining GAF scale scores. Both symptom severity and level of functioning are considered in making specific and more accurate ratings.

In this chapter, we highlight the role of multiaxial evaluation in psychiatric diagnosis. We discuss possible revisions of the multiaxial system. We assert that psychiatry as a medical subspecialty will embrace advances in neuroscience, genetics, and pharmacology. Psychiatry must also incorporate new psychological understanding of temperament, early development, social adversity, coping and adaptation, and subsequent response to stressful events. Twenty-first-century clinicians must communicate a comprehensive understanding of the individual from a multidimensional diagnostic perspective, with the assistance of a multiaxial assessment.

Multidimensional Evaluation

The assumption of a multiaxial evaluation is that the patient will be assessed from multiple dimensions. In a diagnostic assessment, the psychiatrist must consider phenomenological, neurobiological, psychological, and social aspects of the patient. A detailed understanding of the patient allows the psychiatrist to educate the patient, the patient's family, and other clinicians. Treatment must reflect this multidimensional diagnostic understanding. This comprehensive, multiaxial formulation must inform decisions about inpatient and outpatient treatment as well as assessment of outcome.

This approach involves a careful psychiatric diagnostic interview, precise longitudinal assessment of signs and symptoms, attention to critical phases of development, and curiosity about the individual's exposure to stress and subsequent coping and adaptation. The diagnostic interview incorporates a comprehensive mental status examination and cognitive assessment. As knowledge of neurodevelopment grows, clinicians will assess additional risk factors for psychopathology, including exposure to viral illness, brain injury, and perinatal events. Intrauterine environmental distress is increasingly recognized as a risk factor for major brain diseases, such as schizophrenia (Lieberman 1999).

We advocate greater attention to developmental phases and to the occurrence of physical assault, sexual trauma, or persistent emotional trauma at each stage of development. We also advocate that psychopathology during childhood and adolescence be noted, because there will likely be more data about the continuity between childhood and adolescent disorders and subsequent adult psychiatric disorders. The clinician must document the onset and clinical course of disorders as they occur during the patient's lifetime. No comprehensive assessment may omit the effect of substance use and abuse.

Case Formulation

Cases are formulated in the following manner: Using the DSM-IV-TR multiaxial formulation, the clinician carefully applies nosological criteria for diagnosis of a number of categories of illness. He or she recognizes that these categories of illness occur in the context of important personality characteristics. The clinician includes an understanding of the effect of concurrent nonpsychiatric medical disorders. If the clinician continues a multiaxial assessment, he or she notes significant recent psychosocial stressors. Finally, the clinician notes the importance of work and social functioning, in addition to symptoms.

These dimensions of the multiaxial evaluation are regularly embedded in a theoretical framework. Case formulation may lead the clinician to develop treatment plans according to a psychodynamic, interpersonal, cognitive-behavioral, or neurobiological perspective. However, the multiaxial evaluation is a template and is relatively atheoretical as a first step. Regardless of the clinician's theoretical perspective, the multiaxial assessment permits application of empirically based treatment approaches.

Limitations of the Multiaxial Approach

Criticism of the current multiaxial system comes from a variety of sources. Because DSM-IV-TR includes multiple disorders with overlapping symptoms, the problem of comorbidity is not addressed effectively (Frances et al. 1990). In clinical settings, patients routinely meet symptomatic criteria for multiple Axis I conditions (Sargeant et al. 1990). Similarly, patients with personality disturbance may meet criteria for more than one personalty disorder (Widiger et al. 1986). The presence of one or more personality disorders appears to have a considerable effect on treatment of associated Axis I syndromes (Goldstein et al. 1996). Experts in personality disorder diagnosis have emphasized dimensional approaches over categorical approaches. Reviews of the assessment of medical conditions reveal no general taxonomy for the assessment of the relationship between medical and psychiatric conditions (Gruenberg et al. 1997). Using Axis IV in the current multiaxial assessment, clinicians identify recent stressors that affect current presentations. However, limited attention is paid in DSM-IV-TR to early developmental stressors, including early physical, sexual, or emotional abuse. With regard to Axis V in the current multiaxial system, a single rating of functioning—the GAF scale score—is primarily influenced by symptom presentation. Therefore, the Axis V assessment does not involve a specific focus on the importance of work or social functioning as independent factors.

Future Multiaxial Assessment

In emphasizing nosological approaches to diagnosis, Spitzer and Williams (1980) challenged clinicians to improve understanding and communication, minimize diagnostic unreliability, advance neurobiological research, and develop more efficacious treatment. Will a more comprehensive multiaxial diagnostic approach meet these goals? In the twenty-first century, clinicians will face a complex set of conditions in evaluating new patients. We believe that there will be greater attention to earlier manifestations of signs and symptoms of psychiatric disorders, greater understanding of the continuity of these disorders over time, and increased focus on psychological understanding of temperament and its effect on development. The substantial effects of environmental trauma on developing brain function and adaptation must be emphasized (Raut and Stephen 1996). There is increasing understanding of the effect of early developmental and learning disability on adaptation (Silver 1997). Clinicians will evaluate the effects of the following on vulnerability to overt disease: the intrauterine environment; the presence or absence of adequate attachment and bonding in early life; traumatic physical, emotional, and sexual abuse; and chaotic family and social environments (Heim and Nemeroff 1999).

We believe that sophisticated diagnostic understanding will lead to treatment that is empirically based. A nosological approach supports efficacy and effectiveness studies of medications and of diagnosis-specific psychotherapy. The heterogeneity of diagnoses and outcomes necessitates the use of a more detailed and dimensional multiaxial approach.

Future of Multiaxial Diagnosis

In the next decade, multiaxial diagnosis will evolve as clinicians incorporate new sets of information in their diagnostic assessments. Future multiaxial systems will include information obtained because of advances in understanding of the neurobiology and genetics of psychiatric disorders. The following are increasingly relevant to a comprehensive multiaxial diagnostic formulation:

- An understanding of genetic vulnerability. Obtaining a family genetic history will be part of this process. Knowledge of specific genetic markers of vulnerability to psychiatric disorders will also be important.
- A retrospective assessment of the prenatal and postnatal environments, with more careful attention to early neurodevelopment. Studying early neurodevelopment may provide clues to early vulnerability in psychosis and major mood disorders.
- In-depth assessment of psychosocial and family environments during development. Increased research on neurobiological changes associated with early trauma will yield greater information about the effect of abuse on the development of psychiatric disorders (Heim and Nemeroff 1999). This knowledge will permit assessment of current psychosocial stressors as they relate to adaptation to earlier adverse events in a patient's life.
- Objective identification of cognitive and learning disabilities. The ability to identify learning disabilities reliably will also make possible more systematic diagnosis of attentional and concentration difficulties.

The current criteria for Axis I diagnoses will be retained in a future system. Further research on the implications of concurrent Axis I conditions will be required. Comprehensive and reliable assessment of personality disorders consistent with Axis II will also be retained. We support further research on the dimensional aspects of personality and greater attention to early temperamental vulnerabilities, which may be precursors of adult personality disorders.

When consistent and reliable markers of specific mental disorders have been determined through neuroimaging and other research, these markers will become an important component of the general medical axis of the multiaxial assessment. We anticipate that the identification of other non-psychiatric general medical conditions on Axis III will be maintained. This assessment would be similar to the current coding of nonpsychiatric general medical conditions. As psychiatric treatments become more complex through the use of combined pharmacological therapy, there will be a greater need for more vigorous medical assessment involving laboratory testing. Such an approach will cause psychiatrists to be even more attentive to general medical conditions.

Greater understanding of the patient's unique metabolic profile may lead to the development of a treatment axis. Such an understanding would guide pharmacological interventions. For example, an individual might be found to be more sensitive to exposure to specific drugs, and this finding would guide treatment (Seiver 2000).

A more specific measure of social and occupational functioning, one that is independent of symptom criteria, is warranted. An example of this type of measure is the Social and Occupational Functioning Assessment Scale, which is included in Appendix B of DSM-IV-TR.

Also warranted is a more systematic review of a patient's cultural background, as well as an assessment of signs and symptoms that may reflect the effect of cultural differences. Taking cultural aspects into account is an important part of determining a patient's psychopathology.

Coding of a Multiaxial Evaluation in DSM-V

A coding format for multiaxial evaluation in DSM-V is presented in Table 7–1. Additional axes might be included: 1) a neurodevelopmental axis (cognitive or learning disability in youth), 2) a genetic axis (markers of vulnerability to psychiatric disorders or identification of reliable family history data), 3) a pharmacological axis (metabolic markers and unique pharmacological response patterns), and 4) a cultural axis (patterns of experience or behavior that may represent culture-bound phenomena).

Conclusion

The additional domains of information outlined in this chapter could be assimilated into the current system to improve treatment planning, facilitate understanding, and optimize recovery from psychiatric disorders. Clinicians will have a greater diagnostic understanding and capacity to formulate each patient's vulnerabilities, coping style, and response to environmental adversity. We challenge clinicians to assimilate diverse psychological, neurobiological, and genetic data in a future multiaxial format.

TABLE 7–1. Coding format for a multiaxial evaluation in DSM-V

Axis I

Psychiatric disorders

Other conditions that may be a focus of clinical attention

Axis II

Personality disorders

Mental retardation

Temperament

Dimensions of personality

Axis III

Nonpsychiatric general medical conditions

Relevant imaging markers

Axis IV

Psychological and interpersonal stressors

Early traumatic experiences

Axis V

Global Assessment of Social and Occupational Functioning

References

American Psychiatric Association: Diagnostic and Statistical Manual of Mental Disorders, 3rd Edition. Washington, DC, American Psychiatric Association, 1980

American Psychiatric Association: Diagnostic and Statistical Manual of Mental Disorders, 3rd Edition, Revised. Washington, DC, American Psychiatric Association, 1987

American Psychiatric Association: Diagnostic and Statistical Manual of Mental Disorders, 4th Edition. Washington, DC, American Psychiatric Association, 1994

American Psychiatric Association: Diagnostic and Statistical Manual of Mental Disorders, 4th Edition, Text Revision. Washington, DC, American Psychiatric Association, 2000

Frances A, Widiger T, Fyer MN: The influence of classification methods on comorbidity, in Comorbidity of Mood and Anxiety Disorders. Edited by Mosen JD, Cloninger CR. Washington, DC, American Psychiatric Press, 1990, pp 41–59

Goldstein RD, Gruenberg AM, Bruss GS: Co-occurrence of major depressive disorder and personality disorder: treatment implications. Directions in Psychiatry 16:1–8, 1996

Gruenberg AM, Rosenzweig M, Goldstein RD: Axis III: relationship between psychiatric syndromes and medical disorders, in DSM-IV Sourcebook, Vol 3. Edited by Widiger TA, Frances AJ, Pincus HA, et al. Washington, DC, American Psychiatric Association, 1997, pp 401–407

Heim A, Nemeroff C: The impact of early adverse experiences on brain systems involved in anxiety and affective disorders. Biol Psychiatry 46:1509–1522, 1999

Lieberman JA: Is schizophrenia a neurodegenerative disorder? a clinical and neurobiological perspective. Biol Psychiatry 46:729–739, 1999

Raut CP, Stephen A (with Kosofsky B): Intrauterine effect of substance abuse, in Source Book of Substance Abuse and Addiction. Edited by Friedman L, Fleming NF, Roberts DH, et al. Baltimore, MD, Williams & Wilkins, 1996, pp 269–287

Sargeant JK, Bruce ML, Florio LP, et al: Factors associated with 1-year outcome of major depression in the community. Arch Gen Psychiatry 47:519–526, 1990

Seiver LJ: Antidepressant selection in the postgenomic era. Biol Psychiatry 48:875–877, 2000

Silver L: Learning and motor skills disorders, in Psychiatry. Edited by Tasman A, Kay J, Lieberman JA. Philadelphia, PA, WB Saunders, 1997, pp 636–649

Spitzer RL, Williams JBW: Classification of mental disorders and DSM-III, in Comprehensive Textbook of Psychiatry/III, 3rd Edition, Vol 1. Edited by Kaplan HI, Freedman AM, Sadock BJ. Baltimore, MD, Williams & Wilkins, 1980, pp 1035–1072

Widiger T, Frances A, Warner L, et al: Diagnostic criteria for the borderline and schizotypal personality disorders. J Abnorm Psychol 95:43–51, 1986

Williams JBW: The DSM-IV multiaxial system, in DSM-IV Sourcebook, Vol 3. Edited by Widiger TA, Frances AJ, Pincus HA, et al. Washington, DC, American Psychiatric Association, 1997, pp 393–400

CHAPTER 8

Diagnostic Dilemmas in Classifying Personality Disorder

W. John Livesley, M.D.

The classification *personality disorder* remains a troublesome area of psychiatric nosology, despite advances made in DSM-III (American Psychiatric Association 1980) and subsequent editions. The pragmatic approach of DSM-III, which rejected theoretical concepts in favor of traditional clinical categories drawn from diverse schools of thought, created a system that was readily acceptable, even by those who objected to some diagnostic entities. At the same time, the decision to place personality disorders on a separate axis had the desired effect of focusing clinical attention on these conditions. Moreover, the fact that the diagnostic-criteria approach taken was the same as that used with other mental disorders made the system attractive to clinicians and researchers alike. Now, the results of two decades of clinical use and empirical research are challenging the very system that made this work possible.

Clinical application is compromised by poor reliability and the limited value of many categorical diagnoses in treatment planning. Perhaps the most troubling problem for the clinician is the poor correspondence between DSM-IV-TR (American Psychiatric Association 2000) diagnostic categories and typical presentations. The findings of empirical research point to additional problems. Different structured interviews show poor agreement. Statistical analyses of personality disorder criteria and traits fail to replicate DSM concepts, and investigations consistently fail to support the categorical representation of personality phenotypes. The occurrence of major and probably fatal flaws with the system should be neither surprising nor dismaying. The categories and criteria proposed in DSM were never more than arbitrary ideas based on expert opinion. The fact that fundamental revision is now required attests to the success of DSM-III in stimulating research and promoting personality as an integral part of the diagnostic process.

In this chapter, I briefly review the more fundamental problems with DSM-IV-TR before examining the dilemmas that the architects of DSM-V will face if they wish to correct these deficiencies and construct an empirically based system. Taxonomic dilemmas include whether to continue using the current categorical approach or take the evidence into account and incorporate a dimensional structure; whether to continue classifying personality disorder on a separate axis; and whether to use the present diagnoses that are familiar to clinicians or adopt alternative constructs that are more consistent with the evidence and with conceptions of normal personality.

The magnitude of change needed to address these concerns creates a new dilemma: should the system of committees and the consensus-building approach that was used in revising recent editions of DSM be continued, or is a different process necessary for achieving the extensive changes required? After discussing this problem, I consider the kind of alternative approach to classification that is needed to construct a valid system. A two-component structure is proposed that separates the diagnosis of personality disorder from the assessment of personality. With this approach, personality disorder is considered a single diagnostic entity defined by severe self-pathology and chronic interpersonal difficulties that would be classified on the same axis as other mental disorders. A separate axis would be used for recording the individual differences in clinically significant personality characteristics that are important for understanding the way personality disorder is expressed or for managing other disorders.

Problems With DSM-IV-TR

The limitations of the current classification of personality disorder are well documented (Clark et al. 1996; Frances 1982; Frances and Widiger 1986; Livesley et al. 1994; Westen and Shedler 2000; Widiger 1993). Described here are some of the more important problems that need to be addressed.

Limited Clinical Utility

Although the current categorical system is easy to use, it has limited clinical utility. Conditions of actual patients do not match diagnostic concepts very closely, and specific diagnoses have limited value for planning treatment or predicting outcome. Problems arise because most diagnoses are global constructs consisting of multiple traits that may differ in etiology and respond differently to treatment (Shea 1995). This means that knowing a specific DSM diagnosis rarely helps in selecting interventions, because psychosocial interventions are usually directed toward specific behaviors rather than broad diagnoses (Sanderson and Clarkin 1994, 2002). Similarly, pharmacological treatments tend to target specific dimensions such as affective instability, impulsivity, cognitive disorganization, and anxiousness rather than global diagnoses (Soloff 1998, 2000). A different concern about clinical utility is raised by evidence that the conditions of many patients being treated for personality pathology (defined as enduring maladaptive patterns of thought, feeling, motivation, and behavior that lead to dysfunction or distress) could not be diagnosed on Axis II (Westen and Arkowitz-Westen 1998).

Lack of Exclusiveness and Exhaustiveness

The categories forming a satisfactory classification should be mutually exclusive (i.e., should not overlap) and exhaustive (i.e., should exist to classify all cases) (Simpson 1961). DSM-IV-TR has problems in both areas. Multiple diagnoses are the norm (Oldham et al. 1992; Pilkonis et al. 1995; Widiger et al. 1991). The most distinctive category is obsessive-compulsive personality disorder, but even with this category, approximately 70% of cases meet the criteria for a second personality diagnosis (Widiger et al. 1991). This degree of overlap suggests that DSM has not managed to carve nature at its joints. Exhaustiveness is achieved by including the diagnosis personality disorder not otherwise specified (NOS). A catchall category is acceptable if it is used infrequently. In some studies, however, personality disorder NOS is the most common diagnosis. This suggests that the system does not reflect common presentations. These findings present something of a conundrum for DSM-V. Diagnostic overlap implies that DSM-IV-TR contains too many diagnoses (Rutter 1987; Tyrer 1988), and hence fewer diagnoses should be adopted. However, the system does not appear to have sufficient constructs to describe important features of personality pathology. In the later section titled "A System for Classifying Individual Differences in Personality Disorder," I suggest that the solution to this problem is a hierarchical taxonomy of traits in which a large number of specific traits are organized into fewer, higher-order patterns.

Psychometric Limitations

DSM has poor psychometric properties (Blais and Norman 1997). Diagnostic reliability improved considerably with DSM-III, but diagnostic agreement remains a problem even when structured interviews are used (Zimmerman 1994), and agreement across different interviews is modest (O'Boyle and Self 1990). Construct validity is an even greater problem (Livesley and Jackson 1991). Construct validity can be divided into internal validity (the extent to which diagnostic criteria form homogeneous clusters) and external validity (the extent to which diagnostic concepts may be differentiated from one other, and the degree to which they predict external criteria such as etiology and outcome) (Skinner 1981). The internal consistency of criteria sets in DSM-III and DSM-III-R (American Psychiatric Association 1987) was poor, and some criteria were more highly correlated with other diagnoses than with the one for which they were proposed (Blais and Norman 1997; Morey 1988). Internal consistency improved with DSM-IV (American Psychiatric Association 1994), although in DSM-IV and DSM-IV-TR, coefficient alpha falls below the usual criterion level of 0.7 recommended by Nunnally and Bernstein (1994) for histrionic, dependent, and schizotypal personality disorders (Blais and Norman 1997). Blais and Norman (1997) also reported that 9 of the 21 DSM-III-R criteria that were more strongly correlated with other diagnoses than with the one for which they were proposed were retained in DSM-IV and DSM-IV-TR. If these criteria were items on a personality questionnaire, they would be deleted during text construction because they contribute to interscale correlations or, in this case, diagnostic overlap.

Problems with external validity are even greater. External validity has two components: 1) convergent and discriminant validity and 2) predictive validity. Convergent-discriminant analyses are critical tests of a classification. Convergent validity requires that different measurement instruments lead to the same diagnosis. Evidence on this point is variable; different measures show modest agreement (O'Boyle and Self 1990). The biggest problem, however, is with discriminant validity. This requires that diagnoses be distinct from one other and that this distinction hold across different measurement instruments. The extensive diagnostic overlap noted in the earlier section "Lack of Exclusiveness and Exhaustiveness" indicates that diagnostic categories are not distinct. With regard to diagnoses such as narcissistic and histrionic personality disorders and avoidant and dependent personality disorders, criterion discrimination is so poor that it is difficult to differentiate the diagnoses (Blais and Norman 1997). Finally, evidence of external validity is sparse; there is little evidence that diagnoses predict important variables related to etiology and outcome.

Lack of Empirical Support for Diagnostic Concepts

Multivariate studies of personality characteristics consistently fail to generate factors that resemble DSM diagnoses. These findings are obtained whether personality disorder is described using diagnostic criteria (Austin and Deary 2000; Ekselius et al. 1994; Kass et al. 1985) or traits (Clark 1990; Livesley et al. 1989, 1992). Although these findings have not received much attention, they constitute strong negative evidence for DSM-IV and DSM-IV-TR.

Atheoretical Approach

DSM is deliberately atheoretical with respect to etiology. However, it is also atheoretical in the more problematic sense of failing to offer a rationale for selecting diagnoses and criteria. Diagnoses are arbitrary selections drawn from diverse sources, including classical phenomenology (histrionic personality disorder), traditional psychoanalytic theory (histrionic and obsessive-compulsive personality disorders), spectrum disorders (schizotypal personality disorder), object relations theory and more recent psychoanalytic thinking (borderline and narcissistic personality disorders), and social learning concepts (avoidant personality disorder). Given these diverse origins, it is not surprising that the classification lacks coherence or that reliability and validity are poor. More fundamentally, the principles and assumptions leading to DSM's current form are not stated in DSM. What principles led to the placement of personality disorder on a separate axis? What was the rationale for organizing diagnoses into three clusters? What principles and concepts were used to select diagnoses and criteria? The failure to explain the reasons for these decisions makes it difficult to evaluate the consistency with which these principles were applied and to test these assumptions. It also encourages a tendency to overlook negative evidence, because it is not possible to be sure that the underlying assumptions have been fully understood and tested.

Use of Categorical Diagnoses

Many of the problems with DSM arise from the use of discrete categories to classify behaviors that are continuously distributed. This means that clinicians are forced to make arbitrary decisions, leading to poor diagnostic agreement. The use of categorical diagnoses also accounts for great diagnostic overlap, the prevalence of the diagnosis personality disorder NOS, and limited validity. For categorical models based on phenotype, the distribution of clinical features must have discontinuities or points of rarity (Kendell 1975, 1986). These have not been demonstrated for personality disorder. Instead, personality disorders merge with one another and with normality (Frances 1982). Virtually all empirical studies that are relevant to the issue of categorical versus dimensional classification yield findings that are consistent with a dimensional representation of personality disorder (Livesley et al. 1994; Widiger 1993).

Conclusions

An overwhelming amount of clinical and empirical evidence indicates that there are substantial problems with the DSM-IV-TR classification of personality disorder. The magnitude of these problems suggests that they will not be solved by changing criteria sets or adding or deleting the occasional diagnosis, as was done in DSM-III-R and DSM-IV. A new approach is required. The central challenge for the architects of DSM-V will be to develop an empirically based classification that is theoretically coherent with the overall classification of mental disorders, has clinical utility, and satisfies the diverse requirements of an official classification, which include widespread acceptance. The dilemmas posed are taxonomic (in that they concern the contents and organization of the classification) and procedural (in that the extent of the revisions required raises questions about the process through which a new system can be developed).

Taxonomic Dilemmas

Evidence of the poor operating characteristics and minimal empirical support for DSM-IV-TR raises three taxonomic dilemmas for DSM-V: 1) What classificatory concept is most appropriate for classifying personality disorder? 2) Should personality disorders be classified on a separate axis? 3) Are the features of personality disorder best described using the diagnostic concepts proposed by DSM-IV-TR, or is an alternative grouping of clinical features more consistent with empirical data?

Categorical or Dimensional Classification?

Perhaps the most critical decision for DSM-V concerns the taxonomic approach used to classify personality disorder. Other decisions, including those regarding the actual diagnostic constructs used, hinge on this decision. Essentially, the question is whether to retain the categorical model or adopt a dimensional model, or at least incorporate dimensions into the system. This decision has implications beyond the classification of personality disorder because it raises the question of whether the same classificatory approach should be used for all forms of psychopathology. Although DSM has traditionally adopted a uniform approach, it has been suggested that personality disorder and related conditions be classified differently from other disorders. For example, Jaspers (1923/1963) suggested that conditions arising from disease processes be conceptualized as either present or absent and hence classified as discrete categories, whereas personality disorders and neuroses should be classified as ideal types. However, the idea of using different taxonomic constructs for different forms of mental disorder may be difficult for those who revise DSM to accept because the issue touches on a basic assumption of the neo-Kraepelinian approach that provided the conceptual underpinnings of DSM-III and subsequent editions. This approach assumes that there are discrete categories of mental disorder and that there is a clear distinction between normality and pathology (Klerman 1978). The dimensional model questions these assumptions.

Empirical Evidence

The assumption of the categorical model that diagnoses are distinct from one another and from normality is not supported by the evidence (Clark et al. 1997; Livesley et al. 1994; Widiger 1993). As pointed out in the earlier section "Lack of Exclusiveness and Exhaustiveness," there is great overlap among diagnoses, and thus disorders are not distinct. Personality disorder also appears to merge with normality. The distributions of diagnostic criteria in community samples do not reveal evidence of discontinuity between healthy subjects and clinical subjects (Frances et al. 1984; Kass et al. 1985; Nestadt et al. 1990; Zimmerman and Coryell 1990). Similarly, the distributions of personality disorder traits across general population and clinical samples are continuous (Livesley et al. 1992). The disability associated with personality disorder also appears to be continuously distributed. There is no evidence that disability occurs only when a given threshold is reached in terms of the number of diagnostic features present. For example, the risk of anxiety disorders increases as the number of fulfilled criteria for obsessive-compulsive disorder increases, and the risk of alcohol use disorders increases as the number of fulfilled criteria for antisocial personality disorders increases (Nestadt et al. 1990). In addition, impairment as measured with the Global Assessment of Functioning scale associated with personality disorder is continuously distributed (Nakao et al. 1992).

Although the features of personality disorder criteria are continuously distributed, a categorical approach would still be viable if the relationships among these features were different in individuals with personality disorder and those without personality disorder (Eysenck 1987). However, multivariate statistical analyses suggest that the structure of personality disorder traits is the same across samples differing in terms of the presence of personality disorder (Livesley et al. 1992, 1998; Pukrop et al. 1998; Tyrer and Alexander 1979).

These evaluations of the categorical model were based on personality phenotypes. It is possible, however, for the latent structures that are based on discrete genetic or environmental factors underlying continuous phenotypic characteristics to be discontinuous (Waller and Meehl 1998). That is, it is not necessary to demonstrate a discontinuity or bimodality in a distribution in order to have a discrete category or taxon, nor does the occurrence of a discrete taxon preclude dimensionality. Evidence on taxa associated with personality disorder is less consistent than that based on other studies of category-dimension distinction. Using the maximum covariance analysis method proposed by Meehl and colleagues (Meehl 1992; Meehl and Golden 1982), Trull et al. (1990) examined the possibility that a discrete taxon underlies borderline personality disorder criteria. Their results did not support the existence of a taxon. Harris et al. (1994), on the other hand, reported a possible taxon underlying extreme scores on a measure of psychopathy. The issue does, however, draw attention to the problem of compiling a classification from diverse theoretical sources without a coherent rationale. The DSM-IV-TR personality disorders include spectrum disorders, such as schizotypal personality disorder, that may be based on a discrete taxon. Most other disorders, however, appear to represent the extremes of normal personality variants. The issue also draws attention to the lack of an explicit theoretical structure in DSM. Although discrete categories are an assumption in DSM, it is not clear whether they are assumed to be discrete at the phenotypic level or to be based on discrete taxa. This important theoretical and empirical issue must be clarified in DSM-V.

A final line of research that has implications for classification is the genetics of personality disorder. Work on the genetic architecture of normal personality and personality disorder (data were obtained in studies of twins) suggests that a large number of genetic dimensions influence personality (Jang et al. 1998; Livesley et al. 1998). If these initial conclusions are confirmed and personality phenotypes are based on multiple genetic dimensions, each influenced by multiple genes, discrete types in the DSM sense are unlikely.

Advantages and Disadvantages

Although the evidence consistently supports a dimensional representation of personality pathology, there are several advantages to categorical classification that are likely to evoke considerable resistance to change. The approach is agreeable to clinicians: it is easy to use, and categorical diagnoses are easy to communicate. Categorical diagnoses are also consistent with the general approach of medicine and everyday thinking, which relies heavily on categorical concepts. Proponents of categorical classification usually maintain that dimensional systems are more difficult to use. However, many variables routinely assessed in clinical practice, such as blood pressure, are continuously distributed, and this does not appear to pose a problem for clinicians. Empirically derived cutoff scores are used to determine whether a given value warrants clinical intervention. Presumably, it would not be difficult to develop something similar for personality disorder (Frances and Widiger 1986). Another common objection to dimensional structures is the lack of agreement on the basic dimensions of personality. However, as is shown in the later section "Structure of Personality Disorder," there is in fact substantial agreement regarding the basic dimensions of personality and personality disorder.

If a dimensional system were adopted, seven problems with the current classification would be solved, as outlined here:

1. The problem of diagnostic overlap would no longer be an issue. Instead of multiple diagnoses, personality would be represented by a profile of scores on a set of dimensions.
2. The system would have greater clinical utility in terms of selecting interventions, because most interventions focus on specific features rather than global diagnoses. The use of a hierarchical taxonomy of traits would allow considerable flexibility in describing personality.
3. Reliability would increase. The evidence suggests that clinical judgments based on dimensions are more reliable and stable than those based on categories. Reliability would also increase because clinicians could record all important personality characteristics; they would not need to make an arbitrary selection among multiple potentially relevant diagnoses. The amount of information lost would be minimized as a result.
4. The other psychometric properties of the classification would also increase, because most dimensional structures were developed empirically, and associated measurement instruments were developed using the general principles of test construction.
5. Arbitrary distinctions between normality and pathology would be replaced by a graded description that captured more information.
6. A dimensional system would be more compatible with research. Global diagnoses that incorporate multiple constructs are difficult to investigate because the different components may show differential relationships with biological, behavioral, and etiological variables. This means that more subtle effects may not be detected when broader diagnoses are used as independent variables.
7. A dimensional model would integrate the study of normal personality and personality disorder. To date, the classification of personality disorder has tended not to take into account the achievements of research on normal personality. A rapprochement between the two fields would be mutually beneficial (Livesley 2001a).

Despite the obvious advantages of a dimensional scheme, the approach would highlight other problems with the classification of personality disorder. The most important is that the use of dimensions would make it necessary to develop an explicit definition and a set of reliable diagnostic criteria for personality disorder per se. The reason is that an extreme score on a personality dimension is not sufficient for a diagnosis of personality disorder to be made. The important issue is whether the extreme score is clinically significant. This point is discussed in the later section "Definition of *Personality Disorder.*"

Alternative Categorical Concepts

Faced with problems concerning the polythetic categorical approach of DSM-IV-TR and a general reluctance to make a radical shift to a dimensional model, the architects of DSM-V may be tempted to consider alternative categorical concepts. Two possibilities have been discussed: ideal types (Jaspers 1923/1963; Schneider 1923/1950; Schwartz et al. 1989) and prototypes (Livesley 1985; Westen and Shedler 2000). In "Categorical or Dimensional Classification?" I referred to Jaspers's suggestion that ideal types be used to classify neuroses and personality disorders. An ideal type is a hypothetical construct "denoting a configuration of characteristics which, on the basis of theory and observations, are assumed to be interrelated" (Wood 1969, p. 227). In psychiatry, ideal types are idealized descriptions that offer a particular perspective on a condition (Schwartz et al. 1989) and thereby impose conceptual clarity on cases that, by their nature, are fuzzy and imprecise. The assessment process using ideal types does not require the clinician to assess diagnostic criteria and make a diagnostic decision based on the number of features present. Instead, an actual case is compared with ideal or prototypical cases. In the process, the relationship among clinical features is clarified and understood. In some ways, the process is more akin to formulation than to traditional diagnosis.

A related categorical concept is the prototype. Prototypical categories are organized around prototypical cases (the best examples of the concept), with less prototypical cases forming a continuum away from prototypical cases (Rosch 1978). Psychiatric diagnoses show many of the features of prototypic categorization, being inherently fuzzy without clear boundaries between categories (Cantor et al. 1980; Livesley 1985). This structure appears to be especially pertinent to classifying personality disorder, because clinicians seem to use prototypic categorization intuitively in everyday discussion—for example, describing patients as exhibiting "typical borderline personality disorder" or "classic histrionic personality" (Livesley 1985). Clinicians also show high levels of agreement on the prototypal features of

DSM diagnoses (Livesley 1986). Prototypes readily accommodate the fuzziness of personality disorders by establishing gradients of category membership; with monothetic or polythetic categories, by comparison, category membership is an all-or-none matter, rather than a graded quality. Although prototypes resemble ideal types, there are important differences (Schwartz et al. 1989). Prototypes are merely lists of features that define a concept or diagnosis. These lists are not organized, except in terms of the degree to which each feature is prototypical of the diagnosis. In contrast, ideal types are theoretical constructs that incorporate an explanation for the relationship among the features delineating the type.

Westen and Shedler (2000) suggested that the classification of personality disorder would be substantially improved if a prototype approach based on empirically derived prototypes were explicitly adopted. They developed descriptions of prototypes using Q-sort methodology (Westen and Shedler 1999a, 1999b). Clinicians ($n=496$) were asked to evaluate one patient, using 200 descriptive statements developed to represent clinical concepts. Statements were sorted into eight categories according to the degree to which they were descriptive of the person. Q-factor analysis was used to identify clusters or groupings of patients. Q-factor analysis is a type of inverse factor analysis that explores the relationship among subjects, rather than descriptive items or traits as in standard factor analysis. The seven clusters identified were labeled *dysphoric* (consisting of five subtypes), *schizoid, antisocial, obsessional, paranoid, histrionic,* and *narcissistic.* Prototypes of each cluster were then constructed, based on the most highly rated items.

With a prototype-matching approach to diagnosis, clinicians rate the degree to which a patient matches a given prototype. This approach is simpler than assessment using ideal types but provides less information. Westen and Shedler (2000) suggested that this procedure capitalizes on things clinicians do well (i.e., making observations, identifying subtle features that tend to be missed by structured tests, and drawing inferences) and minimizes the use of things that clinicians do badly, such as aggregating and combining data. The proposal certainly capitalizes on the way in which clinicians appear to make decisions. The evidence suggests that they do not combine information about personality disorder as required by DSM (Morey and Ochoa 1989) but rather form opinions based on the degree to which patients resemble clinicians' conceptions of the disorder. For this reason, a prototype-matching approach to diagnosis is likely to be user-friendly. Unfortunately, it is not clear whether prototypes, or ideal types, represent the way personality and behavior are organized in individuals or whether prototypes and ideal types are merely heuristics for organizing clinical information. The prototype method seems to offer a useful way to study how clinicians process information and make decisions. It is unclear, however, that this method is a useful way to study personality. For this reason, ideal types and prototypes are of greater interest in clinical assessment and formulation than in research on the classification, structure, and causes of personality disorder. If ideal types and prototypes were adopted by an official classification, researchers would be forced to use alternative ways to assess personality disorder. This would lead to an even greater schism between research and clinical practice than exists at present.

Conclusions

Empirical evaluations of the category-dimension distinction suggest that an empirically based classification should adopt a dimensional approach or at least incorporate a dimensional scheme to describe individual differences in personality pathology. Although the evidence in favor of the dimensional approach derives from multiple sources, there is likely to be considerable support for the retention of a categorical approach in DSM-V. One reason is that the categorical model has become an enshrined component of the neo-Kraepelinian approach to psychiatry that forms the major conceptual foundation of DSM-III and subsequent editions. As such, it has become incorporated in the assumptions of psychiatry as a profession. The dilemma with regard to DSM-V is whether to 1) adopt a system that is supported by extensive empirical research, and therefore make radical changes to the present system and adopt different approaches to classification in different parts of DSM-V, or 2) retain the traditional model and sacrifice validity.

Separate or Single Axes?

The innovative decision to place personality disorders on a separate axis in DSM-III appears to have been based on pragmatic considerations rather than any theoretical or empirical rationale. The intention was to ensure that personality and personality disorder were assessed during the diagnostic process. However, the simple decision has come to be imbued with more significance. The development of a separate axis created the impression that there are fundamental differences between personality disorder and other mental disorders. This idea encourages discrimination toward those with personality disorder and has led to problems in funding treatment. It is ironic that a decision made to draw attention to personality disorder is often used to refuse treatment and to justify a moralistic attitude toward those suffering from the condition. Given these circumstances, DSM revisers will need to consider whether the negative effects on patients of placing personality disorder on a separate axis outweigh the advantages derived from focusing attention on personality disorder.

There are also sound taxonomic reasons to reconsider this decision. The distinction is similar in magnitude to that made in biological classification between vertebrates and invertebrates. Such major cleavages in a classification should have a sound empirical or conceptual basis. However, major qualitative differences between personality disorder and all other mental disorders are not apparent (Livesley 2001b; Livesley et al. 1994). Moreover, recent evidence suggests that personality disorder shares some vulnerability factors with a range of other mental disorders, such as mood, anxiety, and substance-related disorders.

Phenomenology

Evidence of substantial qualitative differences in phenomenology between personality disorder and all other mental disorders would provide the most convincing justification for placing personality disorder on a separate axis, because the DSM classification is based on phenomenology. The evidence required is not that personality disorder is different from other groups of disorder, such as mood or anxiety disorders (few would dispute this), but rather that the magnitude of the difference between personality disorder and all other forms of psychiatric disorder is such that it warrants a separate axis. The evidence does not support this position. If two groups of mental disorder were to be defined on the basis of phenomenological similarity, it is unlikely that personality disorders would be separated from the rest. Differences between personality disorder and conditions such as somatization, anxiety, and dysthymic disorders are substantially less than differences between these disorders and conditions such as schizophrenia or cognitive disorders.

Assertions of phenomenological differences between personality disorder and other disorders sometimes rely on the argument that the diagnosis of personality disorder is based on traits and attitudes that manifest themselves early in life and remain stable over time, whereas the diagnosis of other disorders is based on symptoms and signs that represent discontinuities in development that fluctuate over time (see Foulds 1965, 1976). Although the idea is appealing, it does not withstand scrutiny. DSM criteria sets for personality disorder are not confined to traits and attitudes but also include items that are similar to Axis I criteria. Consider, for example, the schizotypal personality disorder criteria of odd beliefs and ideas of reference, or the borderline personality disorder criteria of recurrent suicidal behavior and impulsivity. These criteria do not seem different in form from typical Axis I criteria. Moreover, some Axis I criteria are similar to traits. Also, the two axes share dimensions such as impulsivity, affective lability, anxiousness, and cognitive dysregulation (Siever and Davis 1991). Perhaps the greatest problem with the idea, however, is that it confuses personality with personality disorder. Personality obviously differs from psychopathology in the ways Foulds (1965, 1976) suggests, but personality disorder does not. The clinical features of many personality disorder patients fluctuate in severity. Patients with borderline personality disorder, for example, are not always in a crisis. Instead, episodes of instability are often interspersed with periods of more adaptive functioning.

Etiology

Until recently, there has been a tendency to think of Axis I disorders as largely caused by biological factors, and Axis II disorders as psychosocial in origin. If these assumptions were supported by empirical evidence, there would be some validity to using different axes for disorders that differed in etiology. Unfortunately, the origins of mental disorder are more complex. Most conditions, including personality disorder, arise from the interaction of an array of biological and environmental factors. An understanding of the role of psychosocial adversity in the development of personality problems has been supplemented with information about the contribution of biological factors (Siever and Davis 1991), including genetic predispositions (McGuffin and Thapar 1992; Nigg and Goldsmith 1994). Behavior genetic analyses of twin data show that the traits constituting personality disorder, like those of normal personality, have a substantial heritable component (Jang et al. 1996; Livesley et al. 1993, 1998). Heritable traits such as neuroticism that are strongly associated with personality disorder also apparently predispose to a range of Axis I disorders, including mood and anxiety disorders. Far from being etiologically distinct, personality disorder and some Axis I conditions appear to have some etiological factors in common.

Temporal Course

A final reason for asserting that personality disorders should have their own axis is that they are more stable and enduring than clinical syndromes. This argument tends to confuse the stability of personality disorder with the stability of personality traits. Temporal stability is a feature of personality. Indeed, *personality* is usually defined as characteristics that are stable across situations and time. However, the considerable evidence for the stability of personality traits (Heatherton and Weinberger 1994) does not apply to all aspects of personality. Some attitudes, beliefs, and values, including self-esteem, change over time. Many of the features of personality disorder also show considerable temporal instability, and even the presence of the diagnosis fluctuates over time (Barasch et al. 1985; Clark 1992; Mann et al.

1981), probably because of the effects of state factors. As noted in the earlier section "Phenomenology," some cases of personality disorder follow a fluctuating course, with acute symptomatic states and crises and more stable periods. These factors blur the distinction between personality disorder and episodic mental disorders.

A related assertion is that the underlying personality characteristics that give rise to these fluctuations are stable. This is undoubtedly the case, but is this any different from Axis I disorders? Many episodic conditions are associated with underlying vulnerabilities that are similar to those associated with personality disorder (Mayer-Gross et al. 1969). For example, neuroticism or trait anxiety is an enduring trait that predisposes to several Axis I disorders, including major depression (Clark et al. 1994; Rapee 1991). This trait presumably remains once the Axis I disorder has resolved.

Any difference in temporal stability between personality disorder and other mental disorders applies only to episodic mental disorders and not to those that follow a chronic course. Dysthymic disorder, schizophrenia, and some cases of delusional disorder show levels of stability that do not differ appreciably from those of personality disorder. Again, it seems difficult to establish definite distinctions on the basis of course.

Conclusions

As with the decision about categories versus dimensions, the dilemma to be faced during the planning of DSM-V is whether to take empirical and rational evidence into account and use a single axis to classify all mental disorders, or to maintain the tradition of recent editions of DSM by placing personality disorders on a separate axis along with developmental disorders. This has not been the traditional approach of psychiatric nosology. Mental disorders are not separated into two groups in earlier editions of DSM, nor are they separated in most other classifications, including multiaxial systems. If taxonomic principles govern the decision, there is little doubt that a single axis would be used to classify all forms of mental disorder.

Although taxonomic justifications for a single axis are apparent, there are likely to be strong objections to changing the innovation of DSM-III. A common argument is that the use of a distinct axis ensures that personality disorder is not overlooked. This argument, however, confuses taxonomic issues with pedagogic considerations; a classification of mental disorders should ultimately reflect fundamental differences in the way psychopathology is organized. If insufficient attention is paid to personality, this should be addressed through education rather than by introducing a distinction into the taxonomy for which there is little evidence. A related argument is that the prominence that a special place in the nosology gives to personality disorder enhances the likelihood of special attention in terms of research funding and treatment. There is little evidence, however, that these benefits have accrued during the two decades after the publication of DSM-III. In fact, the opposite seems to have been the case. Placement on a separate axis is often used to justify withholding or not funding treatment, and there is little indication that this placement has enhanced research funding.

Current or Alternative Diagnostic Concepts?

The dilemmas just presented concern the structure or organization of the classification rather than the actual diagnostic constructs to be incorporated in DSM-V. It is, however, diagnoses and criteria that are of particular interest to the clinician. Although it is often assumed that a dimensional system would be based on a trait model, current DSM-IV-TR diagnoses could be represented as a set of dimensions (Widiger and Frances 1985). With this approach, each disorder would be rated according to the number of criteria present. This would be the easiest way to incorporate a dimensional approach. Unfortunately, this simple solution is unlikely to be satisfactory, because the evidence suggests that the current diagnostic concepts are inadequate. The frequent use of the diagnosis personality disorder NOS indicates that the system does not capture typical presentations, and diagnostic overlap suggests that current diagnoses do not reflect natural cleavages in the way personality is organized. More convincing evidence that DSM categories are largely arbitrary is provided by the failure of multivariate studies to yield solutions that resemble DSM diagnoses (Austin and Deary 2000; Ekselius et al. 1994; Kass et al. 1985; Mulder and Joyce 1997). For example, Ekselius and colleagues (1994) factor-analyzed DSM criteria for all personality diagnoses (except antisocial personality disorder) assessed with the Structured Clinical Interview for DSM-III-R, Axis II. Twenty-three factors were extracted, most composed of criteria drawn from several disorders. Austin and Deary (2000) also failed to replicate the DSM structure in an item-level analysis of criteria assessed with the same instrument.

Structure of Personality Disorder

Although multivariate studies fail to recapture DSM categories, they consistently identify a four-factor structure underlying personality disorder criteria and traits (Austin and Deary 2000; Livesley et al. 1998; Mulder and Joyce 1997; Presley and Walton 1973; Tyrer and Alexander 1979). For example, Austin and Deary (2000) reported that three- and eight-factor solutions could be justified in their item-level analysis of DSM-IV criteria assessed with the Structured Clinical Interview for DSM-IV. The three-factor solution resembled Eysenck's personality dimensions. Higher-order analysis of the eight-factor solution along with Eysenck's personality dimensions yielded four factors that were interpreted as 1) neuroticism, 2) psychoticism or antisocial, 3) obsessive-compulsive, and 4) suspicious avoidance and introversion.

The robustness of the four-factor solution across studies led Mulder and Joyce (1997) to describe the dimensional structure of personality disorder in terms of the four *A*s: asthenic (personal distress), antisocial, asocial, and anankastic. Other labels used are *emotional dysregulation, dissocial behavior, inhibitedness,* and *compulsivity* (Livesley et al. 1998). This structure is consistently found across studies using DSM criteria and assessments of personality disorder traits. These studies provide strong evidence that four broad factors underlie the domain of personality disorder. Livesley and colleagues (1998) also showed that this phenotypic structure parallels an underlying genetic architecture. Factor analysis of the genetic correlations (as opposed to the phenotypic correlations) among traits delineating personality disorder, using data obtained in twin studies, also generated a four-factor solution that was congruent with the phenotypic structure.

The interesting feature about this structure is that it is consistent with trait models of normal personality. Currently, there is considerable interest in the five-factor approach to personality and personality disorder (Costa and Widiger 1994, 2002). Multivariate studies of normal personality traits consistently identify five major factors or dimensions: 1) emotional stability or neuroticism, 2) agreeableness or warmth, 3) extroversion or surgency, 4) conscientiousness, and 5) culture, intellectance, or openness to experience. These dimensions correspond to personality disorder dimensions of emotional dysregulation (asthenic), dissocial behavior (antisocial), inhibitedness (asocial), and compulsivity (anankastic). Most studies of personality disorder traits fail to find a factor corresponding to culture or openness to experience (Clark 1993). It is not clear whether that is because this domain is not clinically important or because clinicians have simply overlooked its significance and hence it does not appear in descriptions of personality disorder that are the source of traits assessed in multivariate studies. This domain is the one about which there is the least agreement among trait theorists (Digman 1990).

Conclusions

The level of agreement across studies regarding the basic dimensional structure of normal personality and personality affected by disorder is impressive. It suggests that these dimensions, unlike DSM-IV-TR categories, begin to carve nature at the joints and represent fundamental aspects of behavioral organization. Given this evidence, arguments against a dimensional representation of personality disorder on the grounds that different theorists propose different kinds of dimension appear inconsequential. It would seem that any satisfactory evidence-based classification should incorporate these patterns (Livesley 1998; Livesley and Jang 2000).

Procedural Dilemmas

Perhaps the central issue to be faced in developing DSM-V is the extent to which the system will be based on empirical evidence. Although it may seem obvious that a system that is inconsistent with empirical findings will ultimately have little clinical validity or utility, the extensive changes required for accommodating these findings may be difficult to make. What is needed is a new approach rather than a revision of DSM-IV-TR. Medical classifications, however, tend to be conservative, and changes of the magnitude envisioned are likely to elicit considerable opposition. Extensive investment by many individuals and organizations in the present system, and political pressures that are likely to be activated by extensive change, may make it impossible to create a valid structure for DSM-V.

To some extent, this happened with previous editions. When DSM-IV was compiled, extensive evidence that the features of personality disorder were best represented by a dimensional structure was not incorporated. The argument was that a dimensional alternative was not available, and those advocating a dimensional system would be unlikely to agree on major dimensions. The robustness of several critical dimensions and the consistency with which these dimensions are found across different models and studies were simply dismissed. The resistance to change was such that even the suggestion that a dimensional scheme be incorporated in an appendix was rejected.

The evidence for a dimensional representation of personality disorder is now stronger, and there is even greater evidence for the robustness of several key dimensions. Nevertheless, resistance to change continues, and even those accepting a dimensional structure still seem to operate as if an alternative system needs to accommodate DSM concepts; a large number of studies seek to show that DSM diagnoses fit within three- or five-factor models. Given the limited support for the DSM approach, however, it is more important to show that any alternative approach can accommodate the forms of psychopathology that clinicians traditionally consider personality disorder.

These issues raise the following question: What is the most effective way to develop an evidence-based classification? For recent editions of DSM, a consensus-building strategy was used in which revisions were assigned to expert committees whose members represented all shades of opinion, interest groups, and schools of thought. This process generated classifications that were widely accepted. However, the products of committee deliberations were as much sociopolitical statements as scientific documents. As it becomes increasingly apparent that traditional theories of personality disorder are not consistent with the evidence, it is less clear that such an approach will be successful. Different interest groups are likely to resist radical change. It is also not clear that committees of this type will be able to perform the rigorous conceptual analysis and scrutiny of the empirical literature that is required to construct a valid system.

Yet an alternative approach is not readily apparent. The delay that is likely to occur before work on DSM-V commences may help to resolve this problem. Evidence of the limitations of DSM is accumulating to the point that it is difficult to ignore. At the same time, empirical studies are yielding consistent findings that point to some of the essential components of an alternative scheme. When work on DSM-V begins, the outlines of an alternative system are likely to be more apparent than they are now. If this is the case, the usual committee approach may work, provided clear guidelines are established that guarantee that the results of empirical research take precedence over theoretical and philosophical issues and that the resulting system will be subjected to empirical analysis.

Proposal for an Empirically Based Classification

It may be useful to begin a consideration of the possible structure of DSM-V by outlining the requirements of a satisfactory system (Livesley 1998, 2001b; Livesley and Jang 2000):

1. The principles and assumptions underlying the classification should be explicit.
2. The classification should be based on empirical data.
3. The classification should emphasize that personality disorder is a form of mental disorder.
4. The system should be consistent with knowledge in related fields, especially normative personality theory, evolutionary psychology, cognitive science, behavior genetics, and neuroscience.
5. The classification should have satisfactory psychometric properties, and these properties should be specified in ways that facilitate validation.

6. The system should have clinical utility: not only should it be convenient to use, but it should also predict outcome, including response to specific interventions.

Organization: Two-Component Structure

To assess and treat personality disorder, clinicians presumably need a system that enables them to identify clinically useful information and organize this information in a way that facilitates treatment planning. This means that the classification must enable clinicians to determine that they are dealing with personality disorder rather than some other form of psychopathology. This is important because there is abundant evidence both that patients with personality disorder respond to treatment differently than patients with other disorders and that the presence of personality disorder complicates the management of other disorders (Reich and Vasile 1993). Beyond this, clinicians also need a system that enables them to identify differences in personality that are clinically relevant because they have different outcomes or require different interventions.

These simple requirements imply that the classification should have two components: 1) a systematic definition of personality disorder and associated diagnostic items, and 2) a system to describe clinically important differences in personality (Livesley et al. 1994). This structure distinguishes between personality disorder and personality, thereby avoiding problems arising from the tendency to confuse the two. With this arrangement, personality disorder could be classified on Axis I along with all other mental disorders, thereby avoiding the taxonomic and practical problems created by spreading mental disorders across two axes (Livesley 1998; Livesley and Jang 2000). A second axis could then be developed to represent dimensions of individual differences in personality that are clinically important in understanding and managing patients. This axis could be used to describe the different features of personality disorder or clinically important aspects of personality in patients without personality disorder. This would ensure that the relevance of personality to understanding and treating other conditions is not neglected, just as DSM-IV-TR incorporates assessments of psychosocial and environmental problems on Axis IV and general medical conditions on Axis III.

The definition of personality disorder could be developed through a conceptual analysis of the functions of normal personality and the way these functions are disturbed in personality disorder. The diagnostic items developed in this manner could then be revised on the basis of empirical analyses. In contrast, a scheme for representing individual differences should be based on empirical analyses of the structure of individual differences in personality and personality disorder. Ideally, the system would also reflect the genetic architecture of personality.

The diagnostic process based on this structure is shown in Figure 8–1. The first step is to determine whether the criteria for a general diagnosis of personality disorder are met. If this is the case, the diagnostic process continues with the assessment of individual differences. If the criteria are not met, the question is whether personality characteristics are significant in understanding and treating another diagnosable mental disorder. If this is determined not to be the case, the diagnostic process ends as far as personality is concerned. If personality factors are considered important, individual differences are assessed.

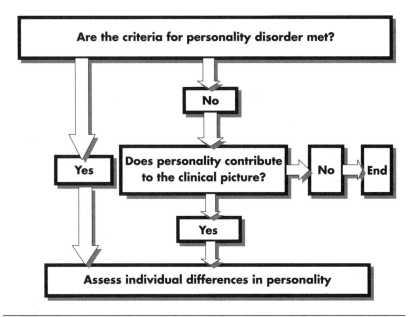

FIGURE 8–1. Diagnostic process using a two-component approach to classification of personality disorder.

The two-component structure incorporates categorical and dimensional constructs. The diagnosis of personality disorder would be recorded as a categorical diagnosis because of the implications for treatment. The characteristics on which this determination is based, however, are continuously distributed; therefore, empirically derived cutoff scores would need to be developed. Individual differences would be recorded as a profile of scores or ratings on a set of dimensions. A similar two-step approach was adopted in the *International Statistical Classification of Diseases and Related*

Health Problems, 10th Revision (ICD-10; World Health Organization 1992). The proposal is also an elaboration of the DSM-IV approach, which extended the DSM-III and DSM-III-R definition of *personality disorder* by offering general criteria for diagnosing personality disorder, in addition to a set of categorical diagnoses to record individual differences in personality disorder. Unfortunately, the general criteria have not received the attention they deserve. Instead, emphasis is usually placed on arriving at a specific categorical diagnosis. The present proposal reverses this situation by placing greatest emphasis on the diagnosis of personality disorder per se. Cloninger (2000) also proposed a two-component approach, in which personality disorder is defined in terms of low scores on any two of four traits (self-directedness, cooperativeness, affective stability, and self-transcendence), and personality is assessed using a series of trait dimensions such as harm avoidance and novelty seeking. The emphasis on diagnosing personality disorder as a single entity, as the first step in the diagnostic process, is also consistent with evidence that the global diagnosis of personality disorder is more stable over time than are diagnoses of specific categories of disorder (David and Pilkonis 1996).

Definition of *Personality Disorder*

To differentiate between personality disorder and personality, and between personality disorder and related mental disorders, a systematic definition of the essential features of personality disorder is needed, one that can be used to develop reliable and valid diagnostic criteria. The simplest definition is that personality disorder represents an extreme position on a trait dimension—that is, it involves either too much or too little of a given characteristic (Eysenck 1987; Kiesler 1986; Leary 1957; Wiggins and Pincus 1989). The implication of such a definition is that personality disorder differs only quantitatively from normal personality. Unfortunately, this idea confuses extreme scores on a personality trait dimension with disorder (Parker and Barrett 2000). As Wakefield (1992) pointed out, statistical deviance alone is neither a necessary nor a sufficient criterion for disorder. In the case of personality disorder, it is difficult to see how an extreme score on dimensions such as conscientiousness, extroversion, or agreeableness is necessarily pathological. Some additional factor needs to be present to justify the diagnosis. DSM suggests two characteristics—inflexibility and subjective distress. Presumably, inflexibility is a function of extremeness (McCrae 1994). Hence, inflexibility is of little additional help in differentiating patients with personality disorder. Nor is subjective distress an adequate criterion; not all individuals with personality disorder are distressed by their traits. Although an extreme level of any trait is insufficient for a diagnosis of personality disorder, it may be possible to identify some dimensions that are particularly important, such as those suggested by Cloninger (2000).

An extension of the extreme-trait definition is Widiger's (1994) proposal, based on the five-factor model, that personality disorders could be diagnosed at the point along the continuum of personality functioning that is associated with clinically significant impairment. Widiger and colleagues (Widiger and Sankis 2000; Widiger and Trull 1991) suggested that clinical significance could be understood as "dyscontrolled impairment" or "maladaptivity" in psychological functioning. This suggestion was made with reference to a general definition of *mental disorder* and hence should apply to personality disorder. The challenge for this approach is to construct criteria to assess "dyscontrolled maladaptivity" reliably. The problem with the approach is that it seems to embrace an ideal concept of normality, because, as Widiger (1994) noted, everyone shows some degree of a maladaptive expression of basic traits. Hence, the distinction between normality and clinically significant impairment would be even more blurred than at present.

The DSM-IV approach to defining *personality disorder* was to adopt the criteria used by ICD-10. Personality disorder is defined as "an enduring pattern of inner experience and behavior that deviates markedly from the expectations of the individual's culture. This pattern is manifested in two (or more) of the following areas: 1) cognition (i.e., ways of perceiving and interpreting self, other people, and events), 2) affectivity (i.e., the range, intensity, lability, and appropriateness of emotional response), 3) interpersonal functioning, [and] 4) impulse control" (American Psychiatric Association 2000, p. 689). In addition, the patterns should be inflexible and pervasive, lead to significant distress or impairment, be stable and enduring, and be traceable to adolescence or early adulthood. The criteria set also specifies that the pattern should not be due to the direct physiological effects of a substance or a general medical condition. The listing of general criteria for personality disorder was a useful development in DSM-IV. The criteria suggested are clinically based and probably acceptable to most clinicians. They are, however, too vaguely worded to translate into reliable measures. They are also arbitrary items that lack a rationale based on an understanding of the functions of normal personality. Instead, they merely catalog features that characterize a wide range of psychopathology. Nevertheless, they serve as a valuable starting point for future classifications.

A different approach is to derive a definition of *personality disorder* from an understanding of the functions of normal personality rather than from clinical descriptions of disorder. The merit of such an approach is that it would bring some coherence to the classification of personality disorder, by integrating it with the study of normal personality and a conception of the adaptive functions of personality (Livesley et al. 1994; Millon 1990; Millon 1996). Cantor (1990) proposed that the functions of personality are best understood in terms of the solution (completion) of major life tasks. These are the tasks or adaptive problems that the person must complete or solve to adapt effectively. Especially important are the universal tasks that confronted humans' remote ancestors in the environment in which they lived as hunter-gatherers. Plutchik (1980) suggested four universal tasks that were basic to effective functioning and survival in that environment: development of identity; solution of the problems of hierarchy (i.e., solution of problems of dominance and submissiveness that are characteristic of primate social hierarchies); development of a sense of territoriality or belongingness; and solution of the problems of temporality (i.e., problems of loss and separation). Adaptive solutions to these tasks are probably equally relevant to adaptation in contemporary society. Solutions to these tasks form core components of personality, and the failure to develop adaptive solutions to one or more of these tasks represents some of the core dysfunctions of personality disorder.

These ideas lead to the notion that personality disorder could be said to be present when "the structure of personality prevents the person from achieving adaptive solutions to universal life tasks" (Livesley 1998, p. 141). This is a deficit definition in that personality disorder is considered a "harmful dysfunction" due to the failure to acquire the structures required to function effectively (Wakefield 1992). This conception could be expressed in more clinical terms, with an evolutionary perspective retained, as 1) failure to establish stable and integrated representations of self and others; 2) interpersonal dysfunction, as indicated by the failure to develop the capacity for intimacy, to function adaptively as an attachment figure, and/or to establish the capacity for affiliative relationships; and 3) failure to function adaptively in the social group, as indicated by the failure to develop the capacity for prosocial behavior and/or cooperative relationships. To complete this definition, it is necessary to add that these deficits are enduring failures that can be traced to adolescence or at least early adulthood, and that the deficits do not arise from a pervasive and chronic Axis I disorder such as a cognitive or schizophrenic disorder. To translate this definition into a set of reliable diagnostic items requires a more detailed description of self and interpersonal pathology (Livesley 1998).

This definition, derived from normative personality theory and evolutionary psychology, resembles clinical concepts of personality disorder. Clinical descriptions typically emphasize two features: chronic interpersonal difficulties, and problems with self or identify. Rutter (1987), for example, concluded that personality disorder is "characterized by a persistent, pervasive abnormality in social relationships and social functioning generally" (p. 454). The psychoanalytic literature, on the other hand, tends to emphasize self pathology, as illustrated by Kohut's (1971) account of the failure to develop a cohesive sense of self in narcissistic conditions, and Kernberg's (1984) concept of identity diffusion that is "represented by a poorly integrated concept of the self and of significant others...reflected in the subjective experience of chronic emptiness, contradictory self-perceptions, contradictory behavior that cannot be integrated in an emotionally meaningful way, and shallow, flat, impoverished perceptions of others" (p. 12). Given the convergence of clinical concepts and the proposed approach to definition, it should not be difficult to develop a reliable set of criteria that are approved by clinical consensus and that can subsequently be refined on the basis of empirical analyses.

As this brief overview suggests, it should be possible for the architects of DSM-V to develop a systematic definition of *personality disorder* that integrates an understanding of the adaptive functions of normal personality with clinical concepts and that captures the complexity and subtlety of clinical ideas without sacrificing reliability. This definition should reflect the essence of personality disorder and the way it differs from other forms of mental disorder. This would improve not only the classification and diagnosis of personality disorder but also the discriminant properties of the overall classification of mental disorders.

A System for Classifying Individual Differences in Personality Disorder

The second component of a classification is a scheme for describing individual differences. As suggested in "Organization: Two-Component Structure," this scheme should probably be based on a taxonomy of clinically important traits that reflects the genetic architecture of personality. There are several advantages to basing a classification on traits rather than other constructs such as defenses, motives, or cognitive structures. The approach would maintain conceptual continuity with the DSM-IV definition of *personality disorder* and with current conceptions of normal personality. Moreover, maladaptive expressions of traits are an important feature of most clinical presentations.

It is often suggested that an obstacle to incorporating traits into a classification is the large number of trait concepts available and the lack of agreement regarding which traits to include. However, as noted in the earlier section "Current or Alternative Diagnostic Concepts?" there is remarkable agreement, across studies of normal personality and personality disorder, on the major dimensions of personality. In fact, this consistency is far greater than the evidence supporting DSM-IV personality disorder categories.

The evidence also suggests that personality traits are hierarchically organized: a large number of lower-order traits are grouped into fewer higher-order traits. For example, agreeableness in the Costa and McCrae (1992) version of the five-factor approach subdivides into trust, straightforwardness, altruism, compliance, modesty, and tender-mindedness. This structure offers a convenient and parsimonious way to incorporate dimensions of individual differences into a classification. The higher-order dimensions provide a broad overview of important components of personality that may be useful for clinical communication and for planning broader aspects of treatment, as well as in some research studies such as epidemiological investigations. However, these broad constructs are not adequate for all classification purposes. Assessment of the lower-order or more basic traits is often essential for detailed treatment planning, because most interventions are not designed to treat broad diagnoses or global dimensions of behavior but rather focus on more specific behaviors of the type presented by the lower-order dimensions (Sanderson and Clarkin 1994). Similarly, studies of etiological and biological processes often focus on more specific components. For these reasons, any taxonomy of individual differences should incorporate this hierarchy.

Higher-Order Patterns

The higher-order factors consistently identified in multivariate statistical studies provide a convenient way to represent broad patterns of personality disorder. Four factors are described (Mulder and Joyce 1997) that may be labeled *emotional dysregulation*, *dissocial behavior*, *inhibitedness*, and *compulsivity* (Livesley 1991; Livesley et al. 1998). These factors, with the exception of compulsivity, describe pervasive patterns of traits that are readily recognizable to clinicians. Compulsivity is less pervasive, and hence it is suggested that this feature be considered a lower-order trait (Livesley 1998; Livesley and Jang 2000).

Emotional dysregulation. Multivariate analyses invariably identify a broad factor characterized by lower-order traits such as affective lability, anxiousness, negative temperament, eccentric perceptions, cognitive dysregulation (the tendency to show cognitive disorganization under stress and to experience brief psychotic symptoms), submissiveness, and self-harm (Clark et al. 1996; Livesley et al. 1998). The breadth of this factor explains much of the overlap among DSM diagnoses. The construct resembles borderline personality disorder but covers a wider range of behaviors, in keeping with the extensive overlap of borderline and other personality diagnoses. The construct is also similar to neuroticism in normative personality theory. The consistency with which emotional dysregulation is identified in analyses of normal personality and personality disorder suggests that this factor should be a central component of any classification of personality disorder.

Dissocial behavior. The second factor identified in higher-order analyses of personality disorder traits is defined by such traits as callousness, rejection (angry, judgmental, and dominant behaviors), and conduct problems. Callousness and rejection appear to be the core features. Traits such as stimulus seeking, narcissism, and suspiciousness often load on this component. This factor resembles psychopathy as described by Cleckley (1976) and Hare (1991). The equivalent dimension in normative personality theory is the negative pole of agreeableness in the five-factor approach, Eysenck's concept of psychoticism (Eysenck and Eysenck 1985), and Zuckerman's (1991) factor of impulsive sensation-seeking.

Inhibitedness. The third factor consistently identified is a pattern characterized by avoidance of intimacy, restricted expression of inner experiences, and social avoidance. This suggests that the essential feature is inhibition expressed as problems in tolerating close relationships, difficulty expressing any kind of feeling, and a reluctance to reveal information about the self. This pattern appears to represent the social withdrawal associated with Cluster A diagnoses and avoidant personality disorder. The pattern also resembles introversion as described by Eysenck (1987) and in the five-factor approach (Costa and McCrae 1992).

These patterns are found consistently across studies, lending confidence to the idea that they describe fundamental differences in the way behavior is organized—that is, they represent "natural kinds" of personality organization. They also appear to describe personality constellations that lead to different interventions and have different outcomes. However, these higher-order patterns are not discrete categories in the DSM sense but rather are broad dimensions that may co-occur. With three patterns, four combinations of extremes scores are possible: emotional dysregulation–dissocial behavior, emotional dysregulation–inhibitedness, dissocial behavior–inhibitedness, and emotional dysregulation–dissocial behavior–inhibitedness. Although these combinations do not closely resemble traditional diagnoses, they appear to capture common clinical presentations. Dissocial behavior–inhibitedness, for example, combines schizoid features with psychopathy, a pattern that is common in forensic settings. Similarly, *emotional dysregulation–dissocial behavior* describes the impulsive, unstable, and reactive behaviors typically associated with many cases of antisocial personality disorder.

These combinations of higher-order patterns are unlikely to include all patterns of individual differences. Personality phenotypes are almost infinitely variable. Some patients who meet the general criteria for personality disorder will probably not exhibit behaviors that are consistent with any of the higher-order patterns. Instead, these patients will show some other combination of specific traits that could be recorded as having a nonspecific pattern, and their personalities could be represented as profiles of scores on the basic or lower-order dimensions.

The hierarchy of personality traits that we are proposing is not complete: not all lower-order traits are part of higher-order patterns. Compulsivity, for example, is a relatively discrete trait that is not strongly associated with other basic traits, and hence it defines a separate factor in higher-order analyses. Because compulsivity is more specific and has a less pervasive influence on adaptive functioning, it is proposed that these behaviors be coded only at the basic level and that higher-order patterns be limited to empirically derived clusters of traits that are associated with considerable degrees of dysfunction.

It could be argued that the higher-order factors are somewhat abstract concepts derived from psychometric analyses that, at first glance, do not appear to match the features of personality that clinicians evaluate when assessing patients. However, the evidence discussed shows that these dimensions adequately explain the DSM-IV-TR personality diagnoses. As noted earlier in the current section, the higher-order patterns also show some resemblance to common DSM disorders: emotional dysregulation resembles borderline personality disorder, the dissocial pattern resembles psychopathy, and inhibitedness resembles the social withdrawal associated with Cluster A disorders. It would also be a mistake to consider the higher-order patterns merely psychometric constructs. They are stable across samples and cultures and appear to reflect underlying genetic dimensions (Livesley et al. 1998), and some of the dimensions that Siever and Davis (1991) suggested link Axes I and II. For this reason, these patterns offer an opportunity to establish a classification that reflects essences rather than appearances (McHugh and Slavney 1998).

Basic Dispositional Traits

Although the higher-order patterns are a convenient way to represent personality disorder for many purposes, the classification should include a set of more specific traits, to represent clinically significant individual differences. Most but not all of these basic traits will be included in the higher-order patterns. For this reason, provision must be made to record them independently of the higher-order patterns. The lower-order or basic-trait level is in many ways primary. Behavior genetic studies suggest that personality is inherited as a large number of genetic dimensions that predispose to specific or basic-level traits (Jang et al. 1998; Livesley et al. 1998). In effect, the lower-order traits should be defined to reflect specific genetic dimensions (Livesley et al., in press)—a step that should also help to ensure that the classification reflects essential differences in the way behavior is organized.

Lower-order studies of personality disorder such as those of Livesley and colleagues (1989, 1992) and Clark (1990) show remarkable agreement on the basic traits of personality disorder (Clark and Livesley 1994; Clark et al. 1996; Harkness 1992). The following is a preliminary list of basic traits:

- Affective lability
- Anxiousness
- Callousness
- Cognitive dysregulation
- Compulsivity
- Conduct problems
- Insecure attachment
- Intimacy avoidance
- Narcissism
- Oppositionality
- Rejection
- Restricted expression
- Social avoidance
- Stimulus seeking
- Submissiveness
- Suspiciousness

These traits could be assessed clinically using a small number of items that would be summed to provide a dimensional score. More detailed evaluation for research purposes could be based on a structured interview or self-report scale. The evidence suggests that self-report scales to assess the basic traits are highly reliable.

These traits are highly heritable (Jang et al. 1996; Livesley et al. 1993). They provide one approach for parsing the domain of personality disorder, an approach that can be revised as the understanding of the genetic architecture of personality unfolds. This list does not include self pathology and interpersonal aspects of personality, because these features are included in the general criteria for personality disorder.

Conclusion

The complex and intricate nature of personality pathology presents a major challenge for psychiatric nosology. It is a challenge to identify discrete clusters of behavioral attributes, either categories or dimensions, that are sufficiently replicable across measures and samples to form the basis of an official classification. One of the difficulties is that personality phenotypes are almost infinitely variable. A simple taxonomy that is easy to use may not be able to accommodate the range of phenotypes commonly encountered. Faced with this diversity and complexity, the architects of DSM-V might have to accept from the outset that it may not be possible to achieve an empirically based classification that meets all other requirements of an official classification. Ideally, such a classification would show historically continuity with its predecessor and be widely acceptable to a range of interested parties. Given the magnitude of problems with the current approach, it is improbable that these conditions can be met, at least initially.

There is probably not enough knowledge at present to build a definitive classification. What one can do, and what is needed, is to identify a number of robust diagnostic constructs that can be used to organize information about personality disorder and collect further empirical information—the ultimate hope being to build a theory that also offers a more definitive classification. The ideas proposed provide a framework that could be used to organize empirical knowledge, which could then be used to organize future studies and their findings. An integrative framework is not a substitute for a theory but an important destination on the way to theory construction.

References

American Psychiatric Association: Diagnostic and Statistical Manual of Mental Disorders, 3rd Edition. Washington, DC, American Psychiatric Association, 1980

American Psychiatric Association: Diagnostic and Statistical Manual of Mental Disorders, 3rd Edition, Revised. Washington, DC, American Psychiatric Association, 1987

American Psychiatric Association: Diagnostic and Statistical Manual of Mental Disorders, 4th Edition. Washington, DC, American Psychiatric Association, 1994

American Psychiatric Association: Diagnostic and Statistical Manual of Mental Disorders, 4th Edition, Text Revision. Washington, DC, American Psychiatric Association, 2000

Austin EJ, Deary IJ: The "four As": a common framework for normal and abnormal personality? Personality and Individual Differences 28:977–995, 2000

Barasch A, Frances A, Hurt S, et al: Stability and distinctness of borderline personality disorder. Am J Psychiatry 142:1484–1486, 1985

Blais MA, Norman DK: A psychometric evaluation of the DSM-IV personality disorder criteria. J Personal Disord 11:168–176, 1997

Cantor N: From thought to behavior: "having" and "doing" in the study of personality and cognition. Am Psychol 45:735–750, 1990

Cantor N, Smith EE, French RS, et al: Psychiatric diagnosis as prototype categorization. J Abnorm Psychol 89:181–193, 1980

Clark LA: Toward a consensual set of symptom clusters for assessment of personality disorder, in Advances in Personality Assessment, Vol 8. Edited by Butcher J, Spielberger C. Hillsdale, NJ, Erlbaum, 1990, pp 243–266

Clark LA: Resolving taxonomic issues in personality disorders. J Personal Disord 6:360–376, 1992

Clark LA: Personality disorder diagnosis: limitations of the five-factor model. Psychological Inquiry 4:100–104, 1993

Clark LA, Livesley WJ: Two approaches to identifying the dimensions of personality disorder, in Personality Disorders and the Five-Factor Model of Personality. Edited by Costa PT Jr, Widiger TA. Washington, DC, American Psychological Association, 1994, pp 261–277

Clark LA, Watson D, Mineka S: Temperament, personality, and the mood and anxiety disorders. J Abnorm Psychol 103:103–116, 1994

Clark LA, Livesley WJ, Schroeder ML, et al: Convergence of two systems for assessing personality disorder. Psych Assessment 8:294–303, 1996

Clark LA, Livesley WJ, Morey L: Personality disorder assessment: the challenge of construct validity. J Personal Disord 11:205–231, 1997

Cleckley H: The Mask of Insanity, 5th Edition. St. Louis, MO, Mosby, 1976

Cloninger CR: A practical way to diagnose personality disorder: a proposal. J Personal Disord 14:99–108, 2000

Costa PT Jr, McCrae RR: Revised NEO Personality Inventory (NEO-PI-R) and the NEO Five-Factor Inventory (NEO-FFI). Odessa, FL, Psychological Assessment Resources, 1992

Costa PT Jr, Widiger TA (eds): Personality Disorders and the Five-Factor Model of Personality. Washington, DC, American Psychological Association, 1994

Costa PT Jr, Widiger TA (eds): Personality Disorders and the Five-Factor Model of Personality, 2nd Edition. Washington, DC, American Psychological Association, 2002

David JD, Pilkonis PA: The stability of personality disorder diagnoses. J Personal Disord 10:1–15, 1996

Digman JM: Personality structure: emergence of the five-factor structure. Annu Rev Psychol 41:417–440, 1990

Ekselius L, Lindstrom E, von Knorring L, et al: A principal component analysis of the DSM-III-R Axis II personality disorders. J Personal Disord 8:140–148, 1994

Eysenck HJ: The definition of personality disorders and the criteria appropriate to their definition. J Personal Disord 1:211–219, 1987

Eysenck HJ, Eysenck MW: Personality and Individual Differences: A Natural Science Approach. New York, Plenum, 1985

Foulds GA: Personality and Personal Illness. London, Tavistock, 1965

Foulds GA: The Hierarchical Nature of Personal Illness. London, Academic Press, 1976

Frances AJ: Categorical and dimensional systems of personality disorder. Compr Psychiatry 23:516–527, 1982

Frances AJ, Widiger TA: Methodological issues in the personality disorder diagnoses, in Contemporary Directions in Psychopathology: Toward the DSM-IV. Edited by Millon T, Klerman GL. New York, Guilford, 1986, pp 381–400

Frances AJ, Clarkin J, Gilmore M, et al: Reliability of criteria for borderline personality disorder: a comparison of DSM-III and the diagnostic interview for borderline patients. Am J Psychiatry 42:591–596, 1984

Hare RD: Manual for the Hare Psychopathy Checklist–Revised. Toronto, ON, Multi-Health Systems, 1991

Harkness AR: Fundamental topics in the personality disorders: candidate trait dimensions from the lower regions of the hierarchy. Psychol Assess 4:251–259, 1992

Harris HT, Rice ME, Quinsey VL: Psychology as a taxon: evidence that psychopaths are a discrete class. J Consult Clin Psychol 62:387–397, 1994

Heatherton TF, Weinberger JL (eds): Can Personality Change? Washington, DC, American Psychological Association, 1994

Jang KL, Livesley WJ, Vernon PA, et al: Heritability of personality disorder traits: a twin study. Acta Psychiatr Scand 94:438–444, 1996

Jang KL, McCrae RR, Angleitner A, et al: Heritability of facet-level traits in a cross-cultural twin study: support for a hierarchical model of personality. J Pers Soc Psychol 74:1556–1565, 1998

Jaspers K: General Psychopathology (1923). Translated by Hoenig J, Hamilton MW. Chicago, IL, University of Chicago Press, 1963

Kass F, Skodol A, Charles E, et al: Scaled ratings of DSM-III personality disorders. Am J Psychiatry 142:627–630, 1985

Kendell RE: The Role of Diagnosis in Psychiatry. Oxford, UK, Blackwell Scientific, 1975

Kendell RE: What are mental disorders? in Issues in Psychiatric Classification: Science, Practice, and Social Policy. Edited by Freedman AM, Brotman R, Silverman I, et al. New York, Human Sciences Press, 1986, pp 23–45

Kernberg O: Severe Personality Disorders. New Haven, CT, Yale University Press, 1989

Kiesler DJ: The 1982 interpersonal circle: an analysis of DSM-III personality disorders, in Contemporary Directions in Psychopathology: Toward the DSM-IV. Edited by Millon T, Klerman GL. New York, Guilford, 1986, pp 571–597

Klerman GL: The evolution of a scientific nosology, in Schizophrenia: Science and Practice. Edited by Shersow JC. Cambridge, MA, Harvard University Press, 1978, pp 99–121

Kohut H: The Analysis of the Self. New York, International Universitites Press, 1971

Leary T: Interpersonal Diagnosis of Personality: A Functional Theory and Methodology for Personality Evaluation. New York, Ronald Press, 1957

Livesley WJ: The classification of personality disorder, I: the choice of category concept. Can J Psychiatry 30:353–358, 1985

Livesley WJ: Trait and behavioral prototypes of personality disorder. Am J Psychiatry 143:728–732, 1986

Livesley WJ: Classifying personality disorders: ideal types, prototypes, or dimensions? J Personal Disord 5:52–59, 1991

Livesley WJ: Suggestions for a framework for an empirically based classification of personality disorder. Can J Psychiatry 43:137–147, 1998

Livesley WJ: Commentary on reconceptualizing personality disorder categories using trait dimensions. J Pers 69:277–286, 2001a

Livesley WJ: Conceptual and taxonomic issues, in Handbook of Personality Disorders: Theory, Research, and Treatment. Edited by Livesley WJ. New York, Guilford, 2001b, pp 3–38

Livesley WJ, Jackson DN: Construct validity and the classification of personality disorders, in DSM-III-R Axis II: Perspectives on Validity. Edited by Oldham J. Washington, DC, American Psychiatric Association, 1991, pp 3–22

Livesley WJ, Jang KL: Toward an empirically based classification of personality disorder. J Personal Disord 14:137–151, 2000

Livesley WJ, Jackson DN, Schroeder ML: A study of the factorial structure of personality pathology. J Personal Disord 3:292–306, 1989

Livesley WJ, Jackson DN, Schroeder ML: Factorial structure of traits delineating personality disorders in clinical and general population samples. J Abnorm Psychol 101:432–440, 1992

Livesley WJ, Jang KL, Jackson DN, et al: Genetic and environmental contributions to dimensions of personality disorder. Am J Psychiatry 150:1826–1831, 1993

Livesley WJ, Schroeder ML, Jackson DN, et al: Categorical distinctions in the study of personality disorder: implications for classification. J Abnorm Psychol 103:6–17, 1994

Livesley WJ, Jang KL, Vernon PA: The phenotypic and genetic architecture of traits delineating personality disorder. Arch Gen Psychiatry 55:941–948, 1998

Livesley WJ, Jang KL, Vernon PA: The genetic basis of personality structure, in Comprehensive Handbook of Psychology, Vol 9: Personality and Social. Edited by Millon T, Lerner MJ. New York, Wiley, in press

Mann AH, Jenkins R, Cutting JC, et al: The development and use of standardized assessment of abnormal personality. Psychol Med 11:839–847, 1981

Mayer-Gross W, Slater E, Roth M: Clinical Psychiatry, 3rd Edition. London, Baillière, Tindall & Cassell, 1969

McCrae RR: A reformulation of Axis II: personality and personality-related problems, in Personality Disorders and the Five-Factor Model of Personality. Edited by Costa PT, Widiger TA. Washington, DC, American Psychological Association, 1994

McGuffin P, Thapar A: The genetics of personality disorder. Br J Psychiatry 160:12–23, 1992

McHugh PR, Slavney PR: The Perspectives of Psychiatry. Baltimore, MD, Johns Hopkins University Press, 1998

Meehl PE: Factors and taxa, traits and types, differences of degree and differences of kind. J Pers 60:117–174, 1992

Meehl PE, Golden RR: Taxometric methods, in The Handbook of Research Methods in Clinical Psychology. Edited by Butcher JN, Kendall CC. New York, Wiley, 1982, pp 127–181

Millon T: Toward a New Personalogy: An Evolutionary Model. New York, Wiley, 1990

Millon T (with David RD): Disorders of Personality: DSM-IV and Beyond, 2nd Edition. New York, Wiley, 1996

Morey LC: A psychometric analysis of the DSM-III-R personality disorder criteria. J Personal Disord 2:109–124, 1988

Morey LC, Ochoa ES: An investigation of adherence to diagnostic criteria: clinical diagnosis and the DSM-III personality disorders. J Personal Disord 3:180–192, 1989

Mulder RT, Joyce PR: Temperament and the structure of personality disorder symptoms. Psychol Med 27:99–106, 1997

Nakao F, Gunderson JD, Phillips KA, et al: Functional impairment in personality disorders. J Personal Disord 6:24–33, 1992

Nestadt G, Romanoski AJ, Chahal R, et al: An epidemiological study of histrionic personality disorder. Psychol Med 20:413–422, 1990

Nigg JT, Goldsmith HH: Genetics of personality disorders: perspectives from personality and psychopathology research. Psychol Bull 115:346–380, 1994

Nunnally JC, Bernstein IH: Psychometric Theory, 3rd Edition. New York, McGraw-Hill, 1994

O'Boyle M, Self P: A comparison of two interviews for DSM-III personality disorders. Psychiatry Res 32:283–285, 1990

Oldham J, Skodal A, Kellman H, et al: Diagnosis of DSM-III-R personality disorder by two semistructured interviews: patterns of comorbidity. Am J Psychiatry 149:213–220, 1992

Parker G, Barrett E: Personality and personality disorder: current issues and directions. Psychol Med 30:1–9, 2000

Pilkonis P, Heape C, Proietti J, et al: The reliability and validity of two structured interviews for personality disorders. Arch Gen Psychiatry 52:1025–1033, 1995

Plutchik R: A general psychoevolutionary theory of emotion, in Emotion: Theory, Research, and Experience. Edited by Plutchik R, Kellerman H. San Diego, CA, Academic Press, 1980, pp 3–33

Presley AJ, Walton HJ: Dimensions of abnormal personality. Br J Psychiatry 122:269–276, 1973

Pukrop R, Herpertz S, Sass H, et al: Special feature: personality and personality disorders: a facet theoretical analysis of the similarity relationships. J Personal Disord 12:226–246, 1998

Rapee R: Generalized anxiety disorder: a review of clinical features and theoretical concepts. Clin Psychol Rev 11:419–440, 1991

Reich JH, Vasile RG: Effect of personality disorders on the treatment outcome of Axis I conditions: an update. J Nerv Ment Dis 181:475–484, 1993

Rosch E: Principles of categorization, in Cognition and Categorization. Edited by Rosch E, Lloyd DB. Hillsdale, NJ, Erlbaum, 1978, pp 27–48

Rutter M: Temperament, personality and personality disorder. Br J Psychiatry 150:443–458, 1987

Sanderson C, Clarkin JF: Use of the NEO-PI personality dimensions in differential treatment planning, in Personality Disorders and the Five-Factor Model of Personality. Edited by Costa PT Jr, Widiger TA. Washington, DC, American Psychological Association, 1994, pp 219–235

Sanderson C, Clarkin JF: Further use of the NEO-PI-R personality dimensions in differential treatment planning, in Personality Disorders and the Five-Factor Model of Personality, 2nd Edition. Edited by Costa PT Jr, Widiger TA. Washington, DC, American Psychological Association, 2002, pp 351–375

Schneider K: Psychopathic Personalities, 1923. London, Cassell, 9th Edition, 1950

Schwartz MA, Wiggins OW, Norko WA: Prototypes, ideal types, and personality disorders: the return to classical phenomenology. J Personal Disord 3:1–9, 1989

Shea MT: Interrelationships among categories of personality disorders, in The DSM-IV Personality Disorders. Edited by Livesley WJ. New York, Guilford, 1995, pp 397–406

Siever LJ, Davis KL: A psychobiological perspective on the personality disorders. Am J Psychiatry 148:1647–1658, 1991

Simpson CG: Principles of Animal Taxonomy. New York, Columbia University Press, 1961

Skinner HA: Toward the integration of classification theory and methods. J Abnorm Psychol 90:68–87, 1981

Soloff PH: Algorithms for pharmacological treatment of personality dimensions: symptom specific treatments for cognitive-perceptual, affective, and impulsive-behavioral dysregulation. Bull Menninger Clin 62:195–214, 1998

Soloff PH: Psychopharmacology of borderline personality disorder. Psychiatr Clin North Am 23:169–192, 2000

Tree TJ, Widiger TA, Guthrie P: Categorical versus dimensional status of borderline personality disorder. J Abnorm Psychol 99:40–48, 1990

Tyrer P: What's wrong with the DSM-III personality disorders? J Personal Disord 2:287–291, 1988

Tyrer P, Alexander MS: Classification of personality disorder. Br J Psychiatry 135:163–167, 1979

Wakefield JC: Disorder as harmful dysfunction: a conceptual critique of DSM-III-R's definition of mental disorder. Psychol Rev 99:232–247, 1992

Waller NG, Meehl PE: Multivariate Taxonomic Procedures. Thousand Oaks, CA, Sage, 1998

Westen D, Arkowitz-Westen L: Limitations of Axis II in diagnosing personality pathology in clinical practice. Am J Psychiatry 155:1767–1771, 1998

Westen D, Shedler J: Revising and assessing Axis II, part I: developing a clinically and empirically valid assessment method. Am J Psychiatry 156:258–272, 1999a

Westen D, Shedler J: Revising and assessing Axis II, part II: toward an empirically based and clinically useful classification of personality disorders. Am J Psychiatry 156:273–285, 1999b

Westen D, Shedler J: A prototype matching approach to diagnosing personality disorders: toward DSM-V. J Personal Disord 14:109–126, 2000

Widiger TA: The DSM-III-R categorical personality disorder diagnoses: a critique and alternative. Psychological Inquiry 4:75–90, 1993

Widiger TA: Conceptualizing a disorder of personality from the five-factor model, in Personality Disorders and the Five-Factor Model of Personality. Edited by Costa PT Jr, Widiger TA. Washington, DC, American Psychological Association, 1994, pp 311–317

Widiger TA, Frances AJ: The DSM-III personality disorders: perspectives from psychology. Arch Gen Psychiatry 42:615–623, 1985

Widiger TA, Sankis LM: Adult psychopathology: issues and controversies. Annu Rev Psychol 51:377–404, 2000

Widiger TA, Trull TJ: Diagnosis and clinical assessment. Annu Rev Psychol 42:109–133, 1991

Widiger TA, Frances AJ, Harris M, et al: Comorbidity among Axis II disorders, in Personality Disorders: New Perspectives on Diagnostic Validity. Edited by Oldham J. Washington, DC, American Psychiatric Press, 1991, pp 163–194

Wiggins JS, Pincus AL: Conceptions of personality disorder and dimensions of personality. Psychol Assess 1:305–316, 1989

Wood AL: Ideal and empirical typologies for research in deviance and control. Sociology and Social Research 53:227–241, 1969

World Health Organization: International Statistical Classification of Diseases and Related Health Problems, 10th Revision, Vol 1. Geneva, World Health Organization, 1992

Zimmerman M: Diagnosing personality disorders: a review of issues and research methods. Arch Gen Psychiatry 51:225–242, 1994

Zimmerman M, Coryell W: Diagnosing personality disorder in the community: a comparison of self-report and interview measures. Arch Gen Psychiatry 47:527–531, 1990

Zuckerman M: The Psychobiology of Personality. Cambridge, UK, Cambridge University Press, 1991

CHAPTER 9

Relationship Disorders Are Psychiatric Disorders

Five Reasons They Were Not Included in DSM-IV

David Reiss, M.D., Robert N. Emde, M.D.

Relationship disorders are distinctive, severe, persistent, painful, and dangerous patterns of relationships between two or more people. They may affect any family relationship or the relationship of any two individuals who have been intimately connected for a sustained period. Since the publication of DSM-III (American Psychiatric Association 1980), there has been a gathering of interest in the inclusion of these disorders alongside other psychiatric disorders now located on Axis I or II. Relationship disorders differ in only one respect from the disorders now included in DSM: the clinician must evaluate the pattern of interaction between two or more individuals to reach a valid diagnosis. Such an evaluation ordinarily involves a direct clinical interview of the individuals, as well as any necessary additional testing. Aside from this singular difference from other psychiatric disorders, relationship disorders have features that are familiar to all trained psychiatric clinicians:

1. Relationship disorders have distinctive characteristics that allow them to be classified. Standard approaches to clinical diagnostic interviewing of people in a relationship are being developed, and there are a growing number of widely recognized, clinically useful, standardized tests to aid the clinician (Messer and Reiss 2000).
2. Relationship disorders cause severe impairments in emotional, social, and occupational adjustment. Indeed, in the extreme, these disorders can lead to serious physical injury and death. Violent parent-child and marital relationship disorders carry serious risk of morbidity and mortality (Knutson and Schartz 1997; O'Leary and Cascardi 1998).

191

3. Relationship disorders have a recognizable clinical course. Risk factors for relationship disorders have been well established through research in many countries. Early forms of these disorders are now more easily recognizable, and the prognosis for some types of relationship disorders, if they are left untreated, is becoming clearer (see, for example, Karney and Bradbury 1995).
4. Relationship disorders have well-recognized patterns of comorbidity with other psychiatric disorders, and this comorbidity has significant implications for the course and treatment of both the relationship disorder and its comorbid conditions.
5. Like many other psychiatric disorders, relationship disorders have patterns of family aggregation. For instance, the same strategies of genetic epidemiology that have been so valuable in other psychiatric disorders are now illuminating relationship disorders (Kendler 1996; McGue and Lykken 1992). For example, identical adult twins are more likely to be concordant for marital or parent-child relationship problems than are fraternal adult twins.
6. The etiologies of many relationship disorders, like those of many other psychiatric disorders, include both biological and psychosocial factors. For example, careful studies of autonomic arousal have illuminated mechanisms underlying the persistence of marital discord (Gottman 1994; Gottman et al. 1995).
7. In many cases, relationship disorders respond to specific treatments, which may include individual psychotherapy (Pilkonis et al. 1984), conjoint family therapy (Bray and Jouriles 1995; Pinshof and Wynne 1995), or even, according to preliminary evidence, pharmacotherapy (Barkley 1988; Sabelli 1990; Schachar et al. 1987).
8. Emerging research suggests that specific interventions can prevent relationship disorders (Markman et al. 1993; Olds et al. 1986, 1988, 1998).

Given these compelling similarities between relationship disorders and other psychiatric disorders, why have the successive editions of DSM not included them? Perhaps the most important reason is that inclusion would necessitate revision of the current conventions of psychiatric practice. In many clinical settings, relationship problems are accorded secondary attention with regard to teaching, research, and involvement of medically trained staff in the care of patients. However, as we will show, relationship disorders play a central role in clinical psychiatric practice even though they are often ignored.

Four additional important obstacles must be overcome before wide consensus is achieved on including relationship disorders in DSM. First, criteria for relationship disorders must be established through clinical research. Second, these criteria need to be securely linked to the larger psychiatric nosology. How do relationship disorders fit into the multiaxial diagnostic systems of DSM? What conceptual relevance does this set of classifications have to other sets, such as the personality disorders? Third, systematic field trials are necessary to ensure that practicing clinicians and clinical researchers are able to classify relationship disorders in a reliable manner. Fourth, important clinical, legal, and ethical issues arising from classifying relationships and relationship disorders need to be addressed, if not fully resolved. These four challenges are summarized in Table 9–1.

TABLE 9–1. Challenges to be met before relationship disorders can be included in DSM

Challenge	Practical examples
Establish criteria for relationship disorders	Are persistent but moderate arguments and disagreements between two spouses, in the absence of physical violence, a criterion of marital conflict disorder?
Link relationship disorder classification and the DSM classification system	Should relationship disorders be listed on Axis I or Axis II, should they have their own axis, or should they be part of an expanded Axis IV?
Ensure reliable classification of relationship disorders by clinicians and researchers	Can clinicians be taught to classify relationship disorders in a reliable way? Are there cultural differences in manifestations of relationship disorders?
Address ethical, clinical, and legal problems associated with classification of relationships and relationship disorders	Does providing a relationship disorder diagnosis to patients suppress the strengths and resilience of the relationship? What are the legal implications of classifying an abusive relationship?

Thus, there are five reasons why relationship disorders were not included in DSM-IV (American Psychiatric Association 1994)—one related to current patterns of clinical practice, and four related to practical problems of classification. The conventions of clinical practice, and the intellectual perspectives that they reinforce, are of central importance but are beyond the scope of this chapter. In this chapter we consider each of the remaining points, those summarized in Table 9–1. Because most effort to date has centered on the first of these four concerns, we devote the most attention to that point, discussed in the section immediately following.

Establish Criteria for Relationship Disorders

DSM-IV (and DSM-IV-TR [American Psychiatric Association 2000]) governs the labeling of cases and noncases. Individuals meet criteria for a particular disorder, and a case of that disorder is said to exist. Individuals who fail to meet these criteria, however much they may be suffering, are not said to have the disorder, and a case does not exist. Often, these subsyndromal conditions pose a serious problem for the classification system, because individuals with these conditions show evidence of considerable suffering that endures in the absence of adequate treatment (Judd et al. 1994; Pasternak 1994). There are three driving forces behind efforts to distinguish cases from noncases. First, there is evidence, for some disorders, that defining a syndrome by a constellation of manifestations and by the duration of those manifestations does allow useful clinical distinctions to be made between serious, sustained disorders and more transient psychological states (Kendell 1982). Second, the decision to treat is a dichotomous one: treat versus do not treat. Finally, third-party payers for health care will reimburse providers for costs relating to "cases of illness."

There is no clear evidence that relationship disorders lend themselves more or less than other psychiatric disorders to this nominal approach. Most systems of relationship classification recognize a gradation between mild and severe forms of disturbance (Anders 1989; Zero to Three 1994) However, the current DSM system focuses on distinguishing cases from noncases and does not include continuous dimensions for recognizing gradations of severity. Is there a rational basis for classifying relationship problems as cases and noncases?

Because relationship disorders do not differ fundamentally from other psychiatric disorders, we address the definition of *case* in ways that are similar to those used for other disorders in DSM. First, we provide a fundamental definition of relationship disorders that lends itself readily to explicit criteria and replicable assessment procedures. Second, we examine previous attempts to develop classifications of relationship disorders; here, we examine whether experienced clinicians, through a careful consensus process, describe relationship disorders that conform to our general definition. Third, we examine more formal clinical evidence obtained in systematic quantitative studies of relationship disorders. Do these studies provide clues that manifestations of these disorders do in fact aggregate as antici-pated by clinical consensus? Are these aggregates, or their components, valid indexes of an underlying disorder? Finally, in a research setting, do these data permit us to distinguish among relationship disorders?

Because of space constraints, we examine in detail only two relation-ship diagnoses: marital conflict disorder and marital conflict disorder with physical aggression. They are offered as examples of the range of relation-ship disorders that could be delineated through comparable logic and ac-cumulation of comparable empirical evidence.

Definition of *Relationship Disorders*

Relationship disorders are persistent and painful patterns of feelings, be-havior, and perceptions involving two or more partners in an important personal relationship. They are marked by distinctive, maladaptive pat-terns that show little change despite a great variety of challenges and cir-cumstances. The most carefully studied relationship disorders are those involving heterosexual, married couples, and parents and children. How-ever, this concept embraces other family and family-like relationships, in-cluding unmarried couples, gay couples, and divorced couples who may remain in prolonged and difficult relationships with each other. It also ex-tends to problematic relationships between adult children and their par-ents, to some grandparent-child relationships, and to some relationships between siblings. The concept has been extended to relationships among several members of a family under the same roof. Indeed, progress has been made in characterizing persistent and problematic patterns of relationships among three or more family members (Messer and Reiss 2000; Oliveri and Reiss 1981, 1984). However, we will focus on heterosexual married cou-ples. The research base for dyadic relationship disorders is much stronger than the research base for relationships involving larger family units.

Relationship disorders can be distinguished from a broad range of in-terpersonal difficulties by four prominent features. First, clear, repeated, and fixed sets of painful and destructive patterns of feelings, behavior, and perceptions can be clearly recognized. There is little flexibility or change in these patterns, and the dyad responds to a range of stresses and chal-lenges with the same distinctive and maladaptive patterns. Second, and fol-lowing from the first, the patterns are of long standing and are not responses to recent stressful events or serious challenges. Third, the corro-sive patterns of relationship are unresponsive to supportive features that may occur naturally in the social environment, including religious, social, and family networks. Fourth, there is clear evidence of a major effect of these patterns on psychological functioning, physical health, social adaptation, and/or occupational effectiveness in one or both partners.

Relationship disorders have many features in common with individual psychiatric disorders. However, they have one unique characteristic: they are a feature of a particular dyad. Thus, the clinician must evaluate both members of the dyad; ordinarily, this evaluation includes seeing the members of the dyad together to identify the most salient patterns of affect, behavior, and mutual perceptions. Although one or both members of a dyad with a relationship disorder often meet criteria for Axis I or II disorders, the diagnosis of a relationship disorder should be made independently of these parallel diagnoses. The coexistence of a relationship disorder and an Axis I or Axis II disorder, as they are currently defined, should be regarded as comorbidity.

The following vignette clarifies many of these concepts:

> Mr. and Mrs. B were referred to a psychiatrist by a cardiologist before Mr. B's coronary artery bypass procedure. The cardiologist was concerned that severe marital problems might complicate Mr. B's recovery from surgery. Of note, the cardiologist had received some of his basic training in psychiatry from the consulting psychiatrist; the training had included instruction on how to recognize relationship disorders. The cardiologist had noted that the couple did not seem to be on speaking terms, and Mr. B had confided to the cardiologist that Mrs. B had a serious drinking problem.
>
> Mr. B was 46 and Mrs. B, 41. Mr. B was the second of three boys. His father died suddenly of a stroke when Mr. B was 12, and his mother, fearing the effect on her young sons, concealed her own grief from them until years later. Mr. B's brother died of a rare neurological condition just before the B couple's marriage. Mrs. B was the younger of two sisters. Her mother was a heavy drinker; her condition worsened after Mrs. B's father died suddenly of a heart attack, 10 years after the B couple were married. Concerned about her mother's drinking, Mrs. B suppressed her own feelings about her sudden loss. The couple has two teenage daughters and a son in fifth grade.
>
> Serious troubles in the marriage began after the death of Mrs. B's father, to whom she had felt quite attached. Mr. B had grown close to him as well, evidently viewing him as a replacement for his father. Instead of grieving, however, he became angry at Mrs. B's preoccupation with her mother's alcoholism. Mrs. B would defend her concerns about her mother and accuse Mr. B of being cruel. Many long arguments ensued, culminating one evening in a severe beating of Mrs. B by her husband. They both denied any physical violence before or after that event. After this violent eruption, Mrs. B began to withdraw from the relationship and began drinking heavily herself. Mr. B began a series of affairs, which were regularly discovered by Mrs. B but rarely challenged. Mr. B came to feel that his wife cared little for him, and he saw her as an irresponsible and preoccupied alcoholic individual. Mrs. B thought her husband cruel and cared little about how his affairs, often with work colleagues, humiliated her.

For years, continuing through the time of the referral to the psychiatrist, she felt intensely lonely and often turned to her older daughter for solace. She recently had thoughts of leaving her marriage but was concerned about the effect of a divorce on their son, who was developing severe oppositional behavior at home and conduct problems in school. On learning that he had coronary artery disease, Mr. B started a new and particularly conspicuous affair, and Mrs. B quit her job as a retail sales clerk.

During the initial evaluation of the couple, the consulting psychiatrist noted that Mrs. B mixed a self-condemnatory description of her own drinking with hesitating complaints about her husband's affairs, complaints tinged with both shame and anger. Mr. B remained cold and sealed off from his wife. He never answered her directly but presented his own complaints about her lack of concern for him. He addressed all his comments to the psychiatrist.

Surprisingly, after the first session with the consulting psychiatrist, Mrs. B found herself filled with sad thoughts about her father, and she reported in the next session that she had wept over his death for the first time. Mr. B listened in silence, but the psychiatrist detected clear signs of emotional involvement in his wife's account. Sensing a hidden reservoir of empathy in this seriously estranged couple, the psychiatrist conducted a brief but successful course of marital therapy.

Current Directions in Classification of Relationship Disorders

The interest in classifying, understanding, and treating relationship disorders is worldwide. However, the most intense efforts to develop a nosology of relationship disorders have been in North America. Five of these efforts are especially noteworthy.

First, a consortium of clinical researchers under the direction of Arnold Sameroff, Ph.D., and Robert Emde, M.D., reviewed concepts and data concerning relationship disorders and their associations with behavioral and medical problems in infants and children. This group focused on parent-child relationship disorders in early childhood and on determining how these disturbances became embedded in enduring patterns of psychopathology. For example, the consortium reviewed evidence that children can learn about patterns of relationships from their earliest experiences in parent-child relationships; these patterns or "working models" shape their expectations of and way of conducting future relationships with others, including their own children (Sroufe 1989; Stern 1989).

Second, a closely related and more recent effort has focused diagnostic attention on the interface between psychopathology in early childhood and disturbances in parent-child relationships. A task group of clinicians, under the auspices of Zero to Three: National Center for Infants, Toddlers and Families, developed a multiaxial classification system for the delineation of disorders as they appear from infancy through age 3. This system, known as DC: 0–3, was published in 1994 (Zero to Three 1994) and is in widespread use in the United States and Europe. It is useful for organizing knowledge, for communicating, and for focusing treatment services. Zero to Three developed a two-axis classification system. Axis I delineates mood, affective, and regulatory disorders as they appear from infancy through age 3. Axis II consists entirely of parent-child relationship disorders and reflects a broad clinical consensus among clinicians working with very young children, in that not only is the parent-child relationship a primary focus of assessment (Bowlby 1988; Cicchetti 1987; Sameroff and Emde 1989) but relationship disorders are often the focus of therapeutic work (Fraiberg et al. 1980; Lieberman 1985). Table 9–2 is a summary of Axis II from this proposal.

Third, a coalition of family therapists and researchers, the Coalition on Family Diagnosis, attempted to achieve a broad consensus on relationship classification among representatives of 15 professional organizations, groups that ran the full gamut of health professionals working with families (Kaslow 1996). Their efforts centered on reconciling the DSM-III-R (American Psychiatric Association 1987) classification system with a broad range of research and clinical experience with families. They made three critical distinctions: 1) Some relationship disorders stand alone and deserve a special classification of their own. Some of these disorders may have associated psychopathology, in which case the disorders of individuals must be separately classified and addressed in a treatment plan. These relationship disorders may also stand alone if there is no classifiable psychopathology. 2) For some disorders, such as forms of depression in adults and conduct disorder in children, relationship data are required for accurate clinical presentation. 3) Finally, some disorders can be defined as individual disorders. However, many of these individual problems (e.g., some eating disorders or depression in adolescents or, many times, schizophrenia and depression in adults) are exquisitely sensitive to problems and disorders in the patient's relationship with a significant other (e.g., a mother, spouse, or child).

Fourth, the Committee on the Family, of the Group for the Advancement of Psychiatry (GAP) (1995), proposed a comprehensive model for the classification of relationship disorders. This was the first effort to advance a nosology that embraces relationship disorders that involve only adults as well as relationship disorders involving both children and adults. This nosology was formulated so that it might be fully included in DSM. Its basic structure is elegantly simple and features two major divisions. First are disorders within one generation, such as marital disorders and sibling relationship disorders. Second are disorders involving two generations; these disorders include relationship problems between parents and children and

TABLE 9–2. Summary of classification of parent-child disorders

Parent-child classification	Clinical manifestation example		Psychological involvement
	Behavioral quality	Affective tone	
Overinvolved	Parent interferes, dominates, and demands while infant is unfocused or submissive	Parent is alternately anxious, depressed, or angry when infant is passive, obstinate, or whiny	Parent eroticizes or romanticizes infant without sense of infant's uniqueness or separateness
Underinvolved	Parent fails to protect infant from danger or to comfort or respond to infant cues	Parent and infant are constricted, withdrawn, sad, and flat	Parent is unaware of infant's needs and may have been neglected as a child
Anxious/Tense	Parent is tense and overresponsive to infant's cues; infant is anxious and compliant	Parent and infant show signs of tension, including anxious mood and motor tension	Parent often perceives infant cues as a signal of parent's incompetence
Angry/Hostile	Parent is insensitive to infant demands and handles infant abruptly; infant is often impulsive and defiant	Interaction is angry and tense, with lack of enjoyment and constricted affect in the child	Parent sees child as threatening to control and unnecessarily demanding
Verbally abusive	Parent is blaming and belittling, and infant is constricted or undercontrolled	Parent is abusive; abuse is often coupled with infant's depression	Parent views infant distress as an attack and is often preoccupied with own childhood
Physically abusive	Parent injures child and/or denies child essentials for survival	Parent and infant show anger, irritability, and tension	Parent cannot set limits, and child's development of fantasy is restricted

TABLE 9–2. Summary of classification of parent-child disorders (*continued*)

Parent-child classification	Clinical manifestation example		
	Behavioral quality	Affective tone	Psychological involvement
Sexually abusive	Parent is sexually seductive or overstimulating, and infant exhibits sexually driven behaviors	Parent's affect is labile, and infant is often fearful and anxious	Parent is preoccupied with own needs and shows distorted thinking, and child often shows notable cognitive defects

Source.   Adapted from Zero to Three: *Diagnostic Classification, 0–3: Diagnostic Classification of Mental Health and Developmental Disorders of Infancy and Early Childhood.* Arlington, VA, Zero to Three/National Center for Clinical Infant Programs, 1994, pp. 46–56.

problems between adult offspring and their parents. The parent-child disorders are divided into three broad categories: abuse and neglect, over- or underengagement, and over- or undercontrol. This classification of parent-child disorders overlaps considerably with DC: 0–3.

Finally, the Task Force on DSM-IV grappled with how to include clinical data about relationships in DSM-IV, and in fact, the *DSM-IV Sourcebook*, Vol. 3, includes several comprehensive chapters on relationship problems (Widiger et al. 1997). However, family researchers and clinicians, as well as many child psychiatrists, were disappointed at the marginal use of relationship data in this reformulation of psychiatric classification. The only relational data in DSM-IV and DSM-IV-TR are a series of relational problems given V codes and presented with "Other Conditions That May Be a Focus of Clinical Attention," and a scale to assess relationship functioning, included in "Criteria Sets and Axes Provided for Further Study."

Development of Criteria Through Clinical Research: Marital Conflict Disorders

The clinician encounters troubled marriages in many ways, but four ways predominate. First, a husband and wife recognize long-standing dissatisfaction with their marriage and come to the clinician on their own initiative or are referred by an astute health care professional, as in the case of Mr. and Mrs. B. Second, there is serious violence in the marriage—usually the husband battering the wife—and the clinician is often alerted by an emergency room, by the legal system, or through a similar route. Third, marital difficulties are noted as part of a comprehensive assessment of an Axis I or II disorder (most frequently depression or alcohol or substance abuse) in one of the marital partners. Fourth, marital difficulties are frequently noted as part of a thorough evaluation of a child with a psychiatric problem; in most of these cases, marital difficulties are linked to problems in a parent-child relationship. Clearly, many clinicians would be aided by valid criteria for these marital difficulties. What clinical manifestations suggest that there is an underlying and serious disorder in the relationship, a disorder that would definitely merit treatment?

Relevant clinical research must address a minimum of three questions. First, do manifestations of marital disorder tend to cluster or aggregate in recognizable patterns? If they do, this knowledge might be particularly helpful to clinicians; by noting that several of these manifestations are present, they could distinguish with greater confidence a serious disorder from a more transitory disturbance. Second, are there important distinctions among manifestations of marital disorders? For example, the GAP proposal (Committee on the Family 1995), which we described in "Current

Directions in Classification of Relationship Disorders," distinguishes marital conflict disorders without violence from those with violence. Is the latter merely a more severe version of the former, or is there evidence that marital disorder with violence is distinctive enough to merit a separate classification? Third, what is the clinical utility of making these classifications? For example, does classification help the clinician identify relationship disorders that are likely to lead to an end of the relationship or to serious physical injury of one of the partners? Does classification help the clinician develop a specific treatment plan?

Do Features of Marital Disorders Aggregate Into Recognizable Patterns?

Clinical research on marriages has not focused on defining cases. As with parent-child relationships, the major emphasis has been on defining and measuring continuous dimensions that distinguish problematic from successful relationships. Useful and valid procedures for defining cases require combining or clustering of these dimensions to make meaningful distinctions between noncases and cases and, where appropriate, to distinguish among different types of cases. Recent clinical research does suggest that severely disturbed relationships can be identified by an aggregate of manifestations. We do not have enough information to determine how many of these manifestations must be present for a severe disturbance to be recognized. Nevertheless, if several are present, the clinician is more confident that there is a severe relational disorder. We focus here on findings from longitudinal studies of troubled marriages. Longitudinal studies effectively define characteristics of marriages with sustained difficulties and point to clinical indicators that a relationship is at high risk of deteriorating further if no treatment is instituted. We also emphasize research on the clustering of clinical manifestations and research findings that help distinguish among relationship disorders. Seven criteria for a case emerge from this analysis.

When one observes the couple, one notes a failure of the partners to control anger, contempt, and other negative expressions toward each other (first criterion). One can observe the partners defending themselves against each other's verbal attacks or criticisms or being unresponsive to each other's initiatives (second criterion) (Gottman 1994). These patterns may reinforce each partner's feeling of being flooded with uncontrollable negative feelings about the other partner (third criterion) as well as each partner's stable attributions that the other partner does not care about him or her or that it is better to work things out alone (fourth criterion). We can see many of these features in Mr. and Mrs. B. There is a history of frequent fights capped by an episode in which Mr. B hit Mrs. B (more on this important event later). This was followed by a prolonged period of mutual withdrawal, a pattern that is most obvious in Mr. B in the interview and that is also manifested in the strong belief held by Mrs. B that Mr. B is cruel and humiliating and in the perception by Mr. B that his wife is self-involved and unloving. Additional data suggest that partners' reports of sexual dissatisfaction with each other (fifth criterion) and their experiences of deficits in problem-solving skills (sixth criterion) may also be part of the syndrome (Snyder and Smith 1986). We are not aware of clinical research data pointing to a minimum duration of marital difficulties, information that would help establish a threshold for a case. It is clear that the marital difficulties of Mr. and Mrs. B are of long standing. (The seventh criterion is discussed in the next paragraph.)

Impairment of social or occupational functioning, to an extent that must be estimated by the clinician, is part of the criteria for a number of disorders in DSM-IV-TR, including substance withdrawal, alcohol withdrawal, and many of the paraphilias. The cardiologist who referred the B couple for psychiatric evaluation was concerned about precisely this point: the threat of marital disruption to Mr. B's recovery from major surgery. Indeed, there is evidence that marital difficulties can impair psychological adjustment during recovery from acute medical illness and can impair psychological adjustment to chronic illness. For example, a recent well-controlled study involving a large sample suggested that marital distress may lead to shortened survival among women who are dialysis patients (Kimmel et al. 2000). There is also evidence that marital difficulties can impair a partner's response to stresses such as unemployment, may result in persistent low self-esteem, and may contribute to psychiatric emergencies including suicide (Burman and Margolin 1992; Gove et al. 1983; Segraves 1980). In general, impaired psychological adjustment, physical health, or occupational and social adjustment (seventh criterion) is a regular feature of marital disorders and can be used to characterize them.

The causal links between marital distress and impairments in the spouse are often complex. The impairments may precede marital distress and contribute to its intensification, marital stress may increase the likelihood that a preexisting vulnerability is transformed into a major psychological difficulty, the effect of marital difficulties may not be apparent until partners are under increased additional stress (e.g., face job difficulties or psychological difficulties), and marital distress and impairments in the spouse may arise from a common cause such as a long-standing personality disorder in one or both spouses. For this criterion to be met, the clinician must make a reasonable determination that impaired adjustment is, in large measure, a consequence of marital difficulties.

Table 9–3 is a comparison of these empirical criteria (which are based on clinical research involving longitudinal and clustering methods) and the

GAP criteria. Although the GAP proposal integrates a considerable amount of current research, the actual criteria for the disorders are a matter of clinical consensus; no research findings are advanced to support just the criteria specified. There is considerable overlap between the two sets of criteria. Moreover, a comparison suggests three types of data that are critical for a classification: observed interaction between the partners, the partners' subjective experience of their relationship, and more complex judgments by the clinician that integrate a knowledge of interaction patterns and the subjective distress of partners as the patterns and distress become evident over time. The GAP criteria summarized in Table 9–3 include two features of troubled marriages that have not yet been the focus of longitudinal, clinical research on marriages: the presence of dysfunctional intergenerational coalitions and the prominence of cheating, exploiting, and deceiving. Moreover, the clinical criteria give particular emphasis to interaction patterns in the marriage. In contrast, the use of questionnaires in a research setting allows for careful examination of intrapsychic attributions that each spouse develops of the other, although it is likely that these attributions could be discovered in a clinical interview.

Are There Relevant Distinctions Among Marital Relationship Disorders That Justify Exploration of Separate Syndromes?

There is wide consensus that the most important distinction among marital relationship disorders is the distinction between those with and those without physical aggression. There are two important clinical reasons for making this distinction. First, and most important, marital violence is a major risk factor for serious injury and even death. Although both husbands and wives can be violent with each other, women in violent marriages are at much greater risk of being seriously injured or killed. Second, these marriages—as opposed to distressed marriages in which there is no violence—have distinctive features that suggest that the disorder in the relationship may be qualitatively different and thus deserving of a separate classification.

The Committee on the Family (1995) recommended a nosological term: *marital disorder with physical aggression*. The most pertinent feature of this disorder is physical aggression on the part of one or both marital partners. Physical aggression can include hitting, threatening with a weapon, physical confinement of a spouse, or marital rape. It is almost always accompanied by verbal abuse and severe threats of physical abuse. In accordance with DSM-IV conventions, we define classificatory terms and present criteria using gender-neutral language. However, all experienced workers in this field give emphasis to the special vulnerability of women in violent marriages (Committee on the Family 1995; O'Leary and Jacobson 1997).

TABLE 9–3. Comparison of empirical and consensus-derived criteria for marital conflict disorder

Empirical criteria	Consensus-derived criteria[a]
Interaction patterns between partners	
Partners fail to control anger, and they exhibit other negative affects (*observation*)	Emotional climate is hostile or indifferent
Partners appear defensive in response to potential attacks or are unresponsive to other's initiative in interaction (*observation*)	One or both partners cheat, humiliate, exploit, or deceive the other more than once
Subjective experiences of partners	
Partners feel flooded with negative feelings about each other (*questionnaire*)	No corresponding feature
Partners feel alone and give up working on problems with each other (*questionnaire*)	No corresponding feature
Sexual dissatisfaction is noted (*questionnaire*)	Impaired sexual relationship over 6 months is noted
Deficit exists in problem-solving communication (*questionnaire*)	Partners are unable to communicate effectively
Integrative evaluation	
At least one partner has impairment in psychological adjustment, physical health, or occupational and social adjustment that is temporally related to marital discord (*several methods*)	Alcoholism and depression are listed as associated features
No corresponding feature	Intergenerational coalitions are present

Note. Methods used to ascertain characteristics are given in parentheses.
[a]Proposed by the Group for the Advancement of Psychiatry.

Clinicians evaluating any marriage must assess for actual or potential violence as regularly as they assess for suicide in depressed patients. Some couples will be quite frank in reporting on violent exchanges, but in other cases, the clinician must inquire carefully. Clinicians should not relax their vigilance after a battered wife leaves her husband, because some data suggest that the period immediately following a marital separation is the period of greatest risk for the woman (Wilson and Daly 1993). Many men will stalk and batter their wives in an effort to get them to return or to punish them for leaving. These initial assessments of the potential for violence in a marriage can be supplemented by standardized interviews and questionnaires, which permit more systematic exploration of marital violence (O'Leary et al. 1992; Straus 1979).

Recent clinical research, all focusing on marriages involving violent husbands, has revealed additional features of these violent marriages in contrast to other distressed marriages. In directly observed interactions, husbands are much more domineering, contemptuous, and critical than in distressed marriages without violence (Cordova et al. 1993; Jacobson et al. 1994). Also, during direct observation of couples interacting, both partners show an unusual degree of provocative belligerence and contempt; this is in addition to signs of fear and sadness in the wife (Jacobson et al. 1994). Fear is also very prominent in reports by abused women about their marriages (Cascardi et al. 1995). Husbands have unusual complaints about their marriages as well. In comparison with nonviolent but maritally distressed men, violent husbands are more likely to report making demands on their wives and withdrawal by their wives (Babcock et al. 1993; Holtzworth-Munroe et al. 1998). Violent husbands also report more jealousy and more concerns that their wives will abandon them (Holtzworth-Munroe et al. 1997). These features suggest a marriage dominated by the husband's efforts at power and control born of jealous preoccupation with his wife and the wife's active and passive efforts to protect herself. There was no evidence of these transactional patterns in the B couple; thus, Mr. and Mrs. B's denial of current violence was credible to the consulting psychiatrist. However, an earlier episode of violence was associated with demands for attention by Mr. B and a withdrawn preoccupation by Mrs. B with her own mother's psychological difficulties.

Evidence suggests at least two distinct types of battering husbands. One type of battering husband is likely to have a pattern of antisocial behavior and extreme exposure to family violence as a child and is more likely to get into fights outside the family. When observed with his wife, even during nonviolent episodes, he is unusually intimidating and belligerent, and his wife shows particularly intense signs of fear. One study suggests that this fear is part of the reason wives do not leave these relationships; hence, such a relationship may be particularly dangerous. A second type of battering husband is more likely to show evidence of a dependent personality disorder and does not engage in violence outside the home. Preliminary evidence suggests that battered wives are more likely to free themselves from these relationships. However, such a relationship must still be regarded as very dangerous because the battering the wife receives is often frequent and severe (Jacobson et al. 1996). These data do not justify a further subdivision of marital disorder with physical aggression, but they do call attention to a particularly malignant variant.

Summarized in Table 9–4 are the clinical features of this disorder, falling under the same three rubrics as those in marital conflict disorder: interaction patterns, subjective experiences of partners, and integrative evaluation. To our knowledge, there is no comparison set of criteria developed through broad clinical consensus. Physical violence is the defining characteristic of marital conflict disorder and is sufficient for classification of a relationship. The other features are important for two reasons. First, clinicians who note these features before they discover the physical aggression will have a heightened suspicion about physical violence and will investigate even if the partners are reticent to disclose such a problem. Second, the features that regularly accompany physical violence are much rarer in nonviolent disturbed relationships and thus suggest that this disorder is a distinctive syndrome.

TABLE 9–4. Empirical criteria for marital conflict disorder with physical aggression

---

Interaction patterns between partners

Hitting, marital rape, and/or threatening with a weapon is reported *(husband's and wife's reports)*

Husband is domineering and critical *(observation)*

Unusual degree of provocative belligerence in and contempt for both partners is noted *(observation)*

Wife appears sad and frightened *(observation)*

Subjective experiences of partners

Husband reports that wife withdraws after he is demanding

Husband shows unusual jealousy and preoccupation with wife

Integrative evaluation

Very high risk variant: Husband shows antisocial personality, is violent outside the home, and, in interaction with wife, is frankly intimidating

---

Note. Methods used to ascertain disorder characteristics are given in parentheses.

What Is the Clinical Utility of Classifying Marital Relationship Disorders?

Clinical research supports two very practical consequences of making accurate classifications of relationship disorders. The first is the decision all clinicians face when presented with symptoms of distress: whether to treat or not treat. The second is the question that arises once a decision is made: Does a distinction among relationship disorders determine what treatment or clinical management is appropriate?

To treat or not to treat. Even though effective family interventions for relationship disorders tend to be brief (Bray and Jouriles 1995), they nonetheless represent significant investments of money, time, and energy by the clinician and the family. Responsible clinicians urge treatment only if they think it unlikely that the relationship disorder will spontaneously remit. Only recently have sufficient data been available for the clinical course of untreated marital disorders to be understood. Indeed, as we have mentioned, these longitudinal data draw special attention to the manifestations of marital disorders we have highlighted (see, for example, Gottman 1994; Karney and Bradbury 1995). With respect to marital conflict disorder, recent data on couples who show the features we have discussed confirm that these couples are at much greater risk than couples who do not have these characteristics. Preliminary data suggest that the risk of separation and divorce is more than three times higher among couples with these features over a period of 3 years (Gottman 1994).

There is also information on the course of violent marriages. Data suggest that over time, a husband's battering may abate somewhat, but perhaps because he has successfully intimidated his wife (Jacobson et al. 1996). The risk of violence remains strong in marriages in which violence has been a feature in the past. Because treatment of these dangerous disorders is very difficult, dissolution of the relationship might be regarded as a positive outcome, and prolongation as a continuing source of danger to the battered wife. This is why attention to the characteristics of the batterer is important in the initial clinical description. Battered women married to violent men who are also violent outside the marriage—women who have been exposed to heavy violence inside the marriage and are noted to be especially intimidated in observed interaction with their spouses—are far less apt to disengage from the relationship. Because attention is shifting toward the characteristics of the batterer and away from the nuances of the relationship patterns, it does seem valid, clinically, to regard marital conflict disorder with physical aggression as more than just a variant of marital conflict disorder. The disorder has distinctive features, presents a very different sort of clinical emergency, and will probably require dramatically different treatment.

Distinctions among disorders and selection of treatment. A variety of marital disorder treatments, most involving conjoint therapy with the couple, have been tested in controlled clinical trials and have been shown to be effective (Bray and Jouriles 1995; Pinshof and Wynne 1995). There many be conditions under which analogous techniques can be used for violent couples (O'Leary 1996). However, often the highest clinical priority is protection of the spouse at risk, most frequently the wife. Indeed, some forms of marital therapy, such as supporting assertiveness by a battered wife in the face of her husband's threats, may lead to more severe beatings (O'Leary et al. 1985) or even death.

Link Relationship Disorder Classification and the DSM Classification System

The fundamental logic of DSM-IV is still in flux. In particular, there is continuing debate about its multiaxial armature (Williams 1997). Nonetheless, assuming that most of this basic structure is preserved in DSM-V, a number of considerations suggest that relationship disorders be placed alongside personality disorders on Axis II. There are, of course, some obvious practical reasons for this idea. Because relationship disorders are not medical disorders, Axis III is not a suitable location, and Axis IV and Axis V do not reflect diagnostic classifications. Moreover, Axis I is overloaded. It seems highly likely that some pruning and consolidation of disorders on this axis will occur as knowledge about their underlying pathogenesis increases. Beyond these practical reasons, there are two conceptual reasons for placing relationship disorders on Axis II. First, there is an easily missed similarity between relationships disorders and personality disorders; the latter are the current major denizens of Axis II. Second, recognizing these similarities will help create a more basic and useful definition of Axis II, solidifying the logic and utility of the axis.

Similarities Between Personality Disorders and Relationship Disorders

There are five notable similarities between relationship disorders and personality disorders. First, both the classification of personality disorders and the classification of relationship disorders require the clinician to integrate a great range of patterns of behavior, affect, and cognitions as they are manifested in a variety of settings. In DSM-IV-TR, the clinician is specifically advised that several diagnostic sessions may be necessary for a valid classification of personality disorders, and multiple informants may be needed as well, a stance on clinical observations that, as we have shown here, is also essential to understanding relationships. Indeed, the considerable integrative effort required for accurate classification of personality disorders may explain why a hurried clinician might overlook such disorders or not have time to document them. The same is true for relationship disorders.

Second, the best information currently available is that in severe parent-child and marital disorders, the patterns of affect, behavior, and cognitions are enduring. This is clearly the case in marital disorder with physical aggression, in which patterns of aggression can begin in the dating, premarital phase of the relationship and persist for years until the abused spouse leaves the relationship. Also determined through study of many dimensions of both marital and parent-child relationship patterns, the stability across months and years is very impressive (Huston and Houts 1998; Rice and Mulkeen 1995; Rusbult et al. 1998). Just as personality disorders get their start early in the life of the individual, so do relationship patterns often become established early in the life of the relationship. Note that the B couple (presented in "Definition of *Relationship Disorders*") handled each major crisis with the same pattern: Mrs. B withdrew, often drinking heavily; Mr. B started or intensified an affair; Mrs. B considered him cruel; and Mr. B felt misunderstood and unloved.

Third, both personality disorders and relationship disorders cause severe impairment of psychological and social functioning. However, partners in a relationship are not always aware of the severity or depth of their relationship disorder and often present clinically with another problem such as physical injury to a wife or child. Even when they are aware of something wrong in their relationship, they very typically blame the other partner and cannot grasp the long-standing relational patterns in which each has been involved. In this sense, both personality disorders and relationship disorders hover in the background of more florid psychiatric disorders, because individuals who have the somewhat obscured disorders are only partly aware of them or attribute many of their principal features to other persons in their social environment.

Fourth, both personality and relationship disorders can be viewed as relatively independent of the Axis I disorders with which they are often associated. For example, although alcohol abuse or dependence may influence or exacerbate marital disorders, marital disorders embrace a range of phenomena that cannot be attributed to the addictive features of a partner's drinking behavior, intoxication, or withdrawal. Indeed, considerable conceptual leverage is gained by keeping these two categories of disorders distinct and observing in detail the mechanisms by which they influence each other. For example, some clinical and research evidence suggests that binge drinking by an alcoholic individual, outside the home, may have less of an effect on marital and family process than steady drinking at home, which often perturbs household routines (Bennett et al. 1987, 1988).

Fifth, there is also increasing evidence that relationship disorders and personality disorders are linked developmentally. A good deal of evidence suggests that in the case of young children, Axis II may contain only relationship disorders, as in the DC: 0–3 system. As the individual passes through adolescence and into adulthood, personality disorders also become appropriate classifications. Indeed, in DSM-IV-TR, most personality disorders are recognized as having their roots in childhood and adolescence. There is increasingly persuasive evidence linking parent-child disorders of childhood to both antisocial and borderline personality disorders of adulthood (Oldham et al. 1996; Patterson et al. 1989; Silk et al.1995; Zanarini et al. 1997). The observed association between the two does not suggest necessarily that relationship disorders cause personality disorders. Both, for example, may have common genetic origins (Pike et al. 1996; Reiss 2000).

A Clearer Definition of Axis II

Adding relational disorders to Axis II would clarify the axis conceptually. The current conceptual uncertainty of Axis II is manifest. For example, it is acknowledged in DSM-IV-TR itself that a central concept of Axis II, the concept of clustering personality disorders into coherent groups, is weak: "It should be noted that this clustering system, although useful in some research and educational situations, has serious limitations and has not been consistently validated" (American Psychiatric Association 2000, p. 686). Furthermore, the idea of doing away with the personality disorder "case" and using continuous dimensions of personality dysfunction instead is still a consideration in DSM-IV-TR. Indeed, DSM-IV-TR includes a synopsis of alternative, dimension-based methods for assessing personality and its disturbances. Finally, as much as any other class of disorders, the specific personality disorders are themselves, with little question, still in the birth process: according to the *DSM-IV Sourcebook*, Vol. 2 (Gunderson 1996), "The existing criteria for most of the personality disorders (DSM-III…[and]…DSM-III-R) were derived by a committee that, for the most part, lacked clinical expertise with the disorders and that had virtually no empirical database as a guide" (p. 647).

Including personality disorders and relationship disorders on the same axis would provide a better definition of the axis itself. A redefined Axis II would have disorders with these characteristics: chronicity; complex patterns of affect, cognition, and interpersonal behavior extending across time; often existence in the background of more florid disorders; and the need for more complex assessment using multiple perspectives, including a developmental one. A redefined Axis II might stimulate clinical research focusing on questions concerning both personality and relationship disorders: How do chronic patterns of behavior and relationships become established? Are there factors common to both types of disorders? What maintains the chronicity of these disorders? How do they slip from full awareness in persons who have them? How can clinicians develop stronger treatment alliances with individuals who have these persistent disorders and are not fully aware of or have little insight into them? How might treatment of personality disorders improve relationship disorders, and how might treatment of relationship disorders improve personality disorders?

Ensure Reliable Classification of Relationship Disorders by Clinicians and Researchers

DSM-IV (and DSM-IV-TR) diagnoses are practical only if working clinicians can make classifications reliably—that is, only if two clinicians seeing the same patient reach the same conclusions regarding classification. Likewise, it is crucial that epidemiologists and other researchers be able to train nonprofessional interviewers to make classification decisions reliably. Important research, particularly involving the large samples ordinarily required for solid epidemiological studies, would be too expensive if fully trained clinicians were needed to collect data.

Our descriptions of relationship disorders as a syndrome serve to clarify that both clinicians and researchers must accomplish three interlocked tasks to make an accurate classification. First, they must observe critical interaction patterns between the two people involved. Second, they must discover subjective perceptions that each participant holds of the relationship. Third, they must integrate additional information about the dyad (e.g., in the case of marital conflict disorder, they must judge whether the relationship disturbance has adversely affected the adaptation of at least one partner). Current evidence suggests that well-trained clinicians who are given clear definitions of relationship problems cannot, without training, reach satisfactory levels of reliability (Shaffer et al. 1991). However, with adequate training, clinicians can reliably discriminate disorders from nondisorders, either by conducting structured interviews (Hayden et al. 1998) or by observing typical interactions, such as the wife feeding the couple's young children (Chatoor et al. 1998).

However, even these carefully constructed assessment procedures, coupled with training of clinicians, do not cover the full range of clinical manifestations of relationship disorders. Thus it seems likely that a fundamental assessment procedure for relationship classification will have three parts: 1) standardized settings for evoking and observing interaction within the dyad; 2) questionnaires for each member to delineate his or her individual perceptions of the relationship, including its level of violence; and

3) a structured clinical interview to supplement questionnaires and observations and integrate additional clinical information.

Reliable methods for evoking, recording, and coding interactions in dyads have been carefully reviewed for use by researchers (Grotevant and Carlson 1989) and clinicians (Bray 1995). It is now clear that clinicians can be trained to reliably code family interactions evoked by standard stimuli, such as asking a family to discuss a recent argument. Typically, these discussions are videotaped and coded. Those codings are sensitive to individual differences among families and their responses to treatment (Szapocznik et al. 1991). It is also now clear that videotaping interactions and systematically coding these taped interactions are an eminently suitable approach for population-based epidemiological studies. Two studies, involving national samples in the United States (Reiss et al. 1995) and Sweden (Reiss et al. 2001), showed that most families contacted by research staff will agree to have their interactions videotaped. Coding of these videotaped interactions of population-based samples is highly reliable and valid (Reiss 2000). Valid and reliable questionnaires used for assessing marital and parent-child relationship problems and suitable for both clinicians and researchers were recently reviewed for the American Psychiatric Association (Messer and Reiss 2000). Recent reports suggest that practical assessments combining many of these methods can be designed and routinely conducted in clinical settings (Floyd et al. 1989). However, these assessments can take 2 hours or longer.

The next step in practical assessments of clinical disorders is to integrate the major advances in assessment methodology into a single, relatively brief module that includes a short clinical interview, selected questionnaires, and a sample videotaped interaction evoked and coded in a standardized fashion. This module would need to be adapted for different types of relationships (e.g., parent-infant, parent-toddler, parent–older child, parent-adolescent, marital). These different modules would need to show the same reliability and validity as the component measures themselves. Two crucial steps would follow.

On the clinical side, the clinical utility of adding relationship classifications to other psychiatric classifications would be a focus of research. The two primary issues to be addressed are 1) how well assessment modules discriminate among relationship classifications and 2) how well these modules discriminate between relationship classifications and other psychiatric classifications. Distinguishing between marital conflict disorder and marital conflict disorder with physical aggression is not a very severe test because the defining characteristic of the latter is a pattern of physical aggression that can be detected without an elaborate nosology or battery of assessments. However, the best-developed nosology for parent-child relationship disorders requires, for example, a distinction between underinvolved and angry/hostile disorders. Can a practical, clinical assessment module make this distinction reliably? A closely related question is, Are relationship diagnoses merely individual DSM diagnoses in disguise? For example, is diagnosing marital disorder with physical aggression just another way of characterizing marriages of men with antisocial personality disorder? Current evidence suggests that this is not likely (O'Leary and Jacobson 1997). How is the relationship classification useful in terms of prognosis, treatment, and prevention?

The assessment module should be put to immediate research use. There is a critical need for population-based epidemiology studies with relationships as the sampling units. A representative sample would be composed of dyads (e.g., parent-child pairs or marital pairs). A matter of immediate importance is the significance of the comorbidity of relationship diagnoses with other diagnoses. For example, there is compelling evidence that the genetic risk of schizophrenia, depression, substance abuse, and certain forms of alcoholism is enhanced in individuals with severe relationship disorders and may be suppressed altogether in the context of healthy relationships free of serious disorder (Cadoret and Cain 1981; Cadoret et al. 1983, 1995, 1996; Cloninger et al. 1981, 1996; Tienari et al. 1985, 1994).

Address Ethical, Clinical, and Legal Problems Associated With Classification of Relationships and Relationship Disorders

Many clinicians who are expert in family assessment and family therapy have raised important ethical issues about classification of relationships. These concerns have centered on potential distortions of the clinician–patient relationship, which may be influenced either by the clinical procedures required to make an accurate classification or by the classification itself.

First, clinicians have been concerned that the process of classification unnecessarily changes the clinician–patient role; the "expert" clinician provides help to the "nonexpert" patient seeking it. This may distort a fundamental process of psychotherapy, in which the therapist and the family work as equals, guided by an emerging definition of both the strengths and problems. These strengths and problems are most tellingly expressed in the patient's own language rather than the professional language of classification. The latter may describe the nuances of the relationship poorly or give undue emphasis to its deficits (Gergen et al. 1996).

Second, and closely related, clinicians have expressed alarm that classificatory labels may become a central part of the framework by which individuals and couples define themselves. Here the process of classification and the classificatory terminology may reduce a patient's self-esteem and ability to conceptualize a broad range of positive options. Furthermore, classification and its terminology may diminish the patient's awareness of facets of his or her personality and relationship that reflect substantial resilience. Assessments should be directed more substantially at the patient's strengths, and an effort should be made to challenge rather than diminish the patient's sense of accomplishment and potential (Wolin and Wolin 1996).

These ethical and clinical concerns are not unique to relationship diagnoses but relate also to widely accepted categories well established in DSM. They arise with special force in the domain of relationships, for two reasons. First, a broad range of family therapy methods do focus on family strengths and resilience, and although these methods recognize serious problems in relationships, they subordinate these problems as quickly as possible. This is clearly illustrated in the case of Mr. and Mrs. B. The therapeutic entrée was not the clinician's recognition of the chronic and perhaps life-threatening marital conflict disorder but his detection of a hidden reservoir of empathy in the couple. Second, and closely related, many groups of clinicians who emphasize working with families have justifiably prided themselves on articulating productive, thoughtful, and influential perspectives on clinical disorders. These perspectives, grouped under the rubrics "'systems' perspectives" and "'constructivist' perspectives," emphasize problems in labeling people as sick and encourage the emergence of the family's own account of its difficulties and aspirations. The perspectives have led to many important innovations in treatment and clinical research, while avoiding classification.

We believe these are serious concerns. Although we are clearly urging that relationship classifications be added to DSM, we also believe that the ethical concerns offered in objection should be taken into account during both the elaboration and application of this nosology. As with current individually based nosology, we believe that a clinician's appraisal of a relationship should involve much more than mere classification; it should cover strengths as well as difficulties in the relationship. Moreover, the therapeutic process must be guided by this comprehensive assessment, and the assessment must be continually updated during the course of treatment, to respond to both the clinician's and the family's emerging understanding of the relationship.

A third ethical concern focuses on violence in the family. Relationship classifications may be perceived, rightly or wrongly, as scientific assessments necessarily free from moral judgments. They may be misperceived by patients and by the public as a basis for recommending treatment for an "illness" and thereby absolving abusive patients from moral responsibility for their acts. This may be particularly problematic in the case of abusing spouses or parents, who may perceive a classification as a rationale for their behavior: the behavior is an illness rather than a moral transgression. Thus, they may await a therapeutic triumph rather than acknowledge that their behavior is not only unethical and dangerous but criminal. This ethical concern, along with legal precedents such as the *Tarasoff* case, remind the clinician once again of the limits of classification. This step, classification— which may enhance both clinical recognition of danger as well as research designed to prevent violence in the first place—is only one step of many in the appraisal of relationship disorders. A clinical classification does not mitigate breaking the law and causing emotional or physical injury.

Summary

We have reviewed a considerable amount of evidence concerning the clinical importance of relationship disorders, as well as specific empirical evidence that would help in the establishment of sets of criteria for the disorders. Moreover, we have provided a summary of data on procedures for assessing these disorders, procedures that promise to be reliable, valid, and clinically useful. We have argued that the inclusion of relationship disorders on Axis II will enhance the clarity of the multiaxial DSM system by providing a clearer definition of Axis II. Finally, we have considered some of the ethical problems surrounding classification of relationship disorders. What conclusions are warranted from this review?

We believe that a task force, composed of clinicians and clinical researchers, should be established by the next DSM committee in order to select relationship disorders that are now mostly clearly delineated by clinical research. The task force should have three objectives. First, it should develop a provisional set of criteria for the most clearly delineated relationship disorders. Second, it should develop assessment modules from existing techniques—combining questionnaires, direct observational techniques, and standardized interviews—that are suitable for assessing these disorders. Third, it should supervise field trials for verifying the reliability and validity of both the assessment modules and the classifications they yield. This process would be similar to those used for other sectors of DSM. This enterprise should result in the inclusion of relationship disorders in DSM-V. We can anticipate three remaining reservations about embarking on this course.

First, there will be concern that this move is premature: there are not enough data on either classification approaches or assessment techniques. Of course, this chapter and other literature reviews we have cited indicate otherwise. Perhaps it is most important to recognize that other sectors of DSM are also in relatively early phases of development. They were included in DSM-III through DSM-IV-TR because of their clinical importance, not because of the strength of the research base. We have already discussed the preliminary status of work on personality disorders when they were first included in DSM. Similar comments could be made now about many of the sexual disorders, for example. Indeed, it could be argued that the volume and clinical utility of research on marital and parent-child disorders far exceed the volume and clinical utility of research on personality disorders and sexual disorders. What is needed now is to reconcile that research with the logic and strategy of DSM. It seems sensible to conclude that this reconciliation should occur *while* relationship disorders are being included in DSM, not *before* they are included.

Second, a critique leveled at DSM more broadly is that there are simply too many diagnostic categories already. Moreover, there is a constant worry that ordinary human misery is being recast as a psychiatric classification, resulting in an overextension of the reach of the mental health professions. At this phase in the DSM system, there is unquestionably a need to prune the classification system. Indeed, as the pathogenesis of psychiatric disorders becomes better understood, links among disorders will be discovered that may enable a broadening of some classifications and a reduction in the overall number of disorders. The link between schizotypal personality disorder and schizophrenia is one of many examples. However, it is reasonable to conclude that the problem of the complexity and breadth of the current DSM system cannot be solved by excluding disorders of great clinical importance. A broad segment of the mental health profession must deal directly with relationship disorders to provide adequate clinical services. This segment includes child psychiatrists, particularly those dealing with young children. It also includes all clinicians who work with adults with any of a multitude of major psychiatric disorders, such as alcohol abuse or depression, whose course and treatment are conspicuously complicated by the presence of relationship disorders.

Finally, many argue that DSM ought to be reserved for clear "medical disorders" that have or are likely to have a "biological base." This position does not seem to us consistent with current research. The pathogenesis of many disorders that would appear to meet these "biological" criteria is strongly influenced by the presence or absence of relationship disorders. The expression of genetic influence on the development of schizophrenia and some forms of depression, for example, is exacerbated substantially in the presence of relationship disorders in the family and may be suppressed if there are no such disorders present. Moreover, relationship disorders have very strong biological roots. For example, quantitative, genetic analysis is as useful for understanding the pathogenesis of relationship disorders as it is for understanding the development of other psychiatric disorders; genetic influences on patterns of both parent-child and marital conflict are surprisingly strong (Reiss 2000). Indeed, current research indicates that the understanding of many psychiatric disorders will be enhanced by fitting together biological and social factors that influence their development. The inclusion of relationship disorders in DSM will provide all psychiatric researchers with a set of tools for realizing this central aim of psychiatrists' clinical calling.

References

American Psychiatric Association: Diagnostic and Statistical Manual of Mental Disorders, 3rd Edition. Washington, DC, American Psychiatric Association, 1980

American Psychiatric Association: Diagnostic and Statistical Manual of Mental Disorders, 3rd Edition, Revised. Washington, DC, American Psychiatric Association, 1987

American Psychiatric Association: Diagnostic and Statistical Manual of Mental Disorders, 4th Edition. Washington, DC, American Psychiatric Association, 1994

American Psychiatric Association: Diagnostic and Statistical Manual of Mental Disorders, 4th Edition, Text Revision. Washington, DC, American Psychiatric Association, 2000

Anders TF: Clinical syndromes, relationships disorders and their assessment, in Relationship Disturbances in Early Childhood. Edited by Sameroff AJ, Emde RN. New York, Basic Books, 1989, pp 125–144

Babcock J, Waltz J, Jacobson NS, et al: Power and violence: the relationship between communication patterns, power discrepancies, and domestic violence. J Consult Clin Psychol 61:40–50, 1993

Barkley RA: The effects of methylphenidate on the interactions of preschool ADHD children with their mothers. J Am Acad Child Adolesc Psychiatry 27:336–341, 1988

Bennett LA, Wolin SJ, Reiss D, et al: Couples at risk for transmission of alcoholism: protective influences. Fam Process 26:111–129, 1987

Bennett LA, Wolin SJ, Reiss D: Deliberate family process: a strategy for protecting children of alcoholics. Br J Addict 83:821–829, 1988

Bowlby J: A Secure Base: Parent-Child Attachment and Healthy Human Development. New York, Basic Books, 1988

Bray JH: Family assessment: current issues in evaluating families. Family Relations: Journal of Applied Family & Child Studies 44:469–477, 1995

Bray JH, Jouriles EN: Treatment of marital conflict and prevention of divorce. J Marital Fam Ther 21:461–473, 1995

Burman B, Margolin G: Analysis of the association between marital relationships and health problems: an interactional perspective. Psychol Bull 112:39–63, 1992

Cadoret RJ, Cain CA: Genetic-environmental interaction in adoption studies of antisocial behavior, in Biological Psychiatry 1981: Proceedings of the 3rd World Congress of Biological Psychiatry (Developments in Psychiatry, Vol 5). Edited by Perris S, Struwe G, Jansson B. New York, Elsevier North-Holland, 1981, pp 97–100

Cadoret R[J], Cain CA, Crowe RR: Evidence for gene-environment interaction in the development of adolescent antisocial behavior. Behav Genet 13:301–310, 1983

Cadoret RJ, Yates WR, Troughton E, et al: Genetic-environmental interaction in the genesis of aggressivity and conduct disorders. Arch Gen Psychiatry 52:916–924, 1995

Cadoret RJ, Winokur G, Langbehn D, et al: Depression spectrum disease, I: the role of gene-environment interaction. Am J Psychiatry 153:892–899, 1996

Cascardi M, O'Leary KD, Lawrence EE, et al: Characteristics of women physically abused by their spouses and who seek treatment regarding marital conflict. J Consult Clin Psychol 63:616–623, 1995

Chatoor I, Hirsch R, Ganiban J, et al: Diagnosing infantile anorexia: the observation of mother-infant interactions. J Am Acad Child Adolesc Psychiatry 37:959–967, 1998

Cicchetti D: Developmental psychopathology in infancy: illustrations from the study of maltreated youngsters. J Consult Clin Psychol 55:837–845, 1987

Cloninger CR, Bohman M, Sigvardsson S: Inheritance of alcohol abuse: crossfostering analysis of adopted men. Arch Gen Psychiatry 38:861–868, 1981

Cloninger CR, Sigvardsson S, Bohman M: Type I and type II alcoholism: an update. Alcohol Health Res World 20:18–23, 1996

Committee on the Family, Group for the Advancement of Psychiatry: A model for the classification and diagnosis of relational disorders. Psychiatr Serv 46:926–931, 1995

Cordova JV, Jacobson NS, Gottman JM, et al: Negative reciprocity and communication in couples with a violent husband. J Abnorm Psychol 102:559–564, 1993

Floyd FJ, Weinand JW, Cimmarusti RA: Clinical family assessment: applying structured measurement procedures in treatment settings. J Marital Fam Ther 15:271–288, 1989

Fraiberg S, Adelson E, Shapiro V: Clinical Studies in Infant Mental Health: The First Year of Life. New York, Basic Books, 1980

Gergen KJ, Hoffman L, Anderson H: Is diagnosis a disaster? a constructionist trialogue, in Handbook of Relational Diagnosis and Dysfunctional Family Patterns. Edited by Kaslow FW. New York, Wiley, 1996, pp 102–118

Gottman JM: What Predicts Divorce? Hillsdale, NJ, Erlbaum, 1994

Gottman JM, Jacobson NS, Rushe RH, et al: The relationship between heart rate reactivity, emotionally aggressive behavior and general violence in batterers. J Fam Psychol 9:227–248, 1995

Gove WR, Hughes M, Style CB: Does marriage have positive effects on the psychological well-being of the individual? J Health Soc Behav 24:122–131, 1983

Grotevant HD, Carlson CI: Family Assessment: A Guide to Methods and Measures. New York, Guilford, 1989

Gunderson J: Introduction to Section IV, Personality Disorders, in DSM-IV Sourcebook, Vol 2. Edited by Widiger TA, Frances AJ, Pincus HA, et al. Washington, DC, American Psychiatric Association, 1996, pp 647–664

Hayden LC, Schiller M, Dickstein S, et al: Levels of family assessment, I: family, marital, and parent-child interaction. J Fam Psychol 12:7–22, 1998

Holtzworth-Munroe A, Stuart GL, Hutchinson G: Violent versus nonviolent husbands: differences in attachment patterns, dependency, and jealousy. J Fam Psychol 11:314–331, 1997

Holtzworth-Munroe A, Smutzler N, Stuart GL: Demand and withdraw communication among couples experiencing husband violence. J Consult Clin Psychol 66:731–743, 1998

Huston TL, Houts RM: The psychological infrastructure of courtship and marriage, in The Developmental Course of Marital Dysfunction. Edited by Bradbury TN. New York, Cambridge University Press, 1998, pp 114–151

Jacobson NS, Gottman JM, Waltz J, et al: Affect, verbal content, and psychophysiology in the arguments of couples with a violent husband. J Consult Clin Psychol 62:982–988, 1994

Jacobson NS, Gottman JM, Berns S, et al: Psychological factors in the longitudinal course of battering: when do the couples split up? when does the abuse decrease? Violence Vict 11:371–392, 1996

Judd LL, Rapaport MH, Paulus MP, et al: Subsyndromal symptomatic depression: a new mood disorder? J Clin Psychiatry 55 (suppl):18–28, 1994

Karney BR, Bradbury TN: The longitudinal course of marital quality and stability: a review of theory, method and research. Psychol Bull 118:3–34, 1995

Kaslow FW (ed): Handbook of Relational Diagnosis and Dysfunctional Family Patterns. New York, Wiley, 1996

Kendell RE: The choice of diagnostic criteria for biological research. Arch Gen Psychiatry 39:1334–1339, 1982

Kendler KS: Parenting: a genetic-epidemiologic perspective. Am J Psychiatry 153:11–20, 1996

Kimmel PL, Peterson RA, Weihs KL, et al: Dyadic relationship conflict, gender and mortality in urban hemodialysis patients. J Am Soc Nephrol 11:1518–1525, 2000

Knutson JF, Schartz HA: Physical abuse and neglect of children, in DSM-IV Sourcebook, Vol 3. Edited by Widiger TA, Frances AJ, Pincus HA, et al. Washington, DC, American Psychiatric Association, 1997, pp 713–804

Lieberman AF: Infant mental health: a model for service delivery. J Clin Child Psychol 14:196–201, 1985

Markman HJ, Renick MJ, Floyd FJ, et al: Preventing marital distress through communication and conflict management training: a 4- and 5-year followup. J Consult Clin Psychol 61:70–77, 1993

McGue M, Lykken DT: Genetic influence on risk of divorce. Psychol Sci 3:368–373, 1992

Messer SC, Reiss D: Family and relational issues measures, in Handbook of Psychiatric Measures. Edited by Rush AJ, Pincus HA, First MB, et al. Washington, DC, American Psychiatric Association, 2000, pp 239–260

Oldham JM, Skodol AE, Gallaher PE, et al: Relationship of borderline symptoms to histories of abuse and neglect: a pilot study. Psychiatr Q 67:287–295, 1996

Olds DL, Henderson CR Jr, Chamberlin R, et al: Preventing child abuse and neglect: a randomized trial of nurse home visitation. Pediatrics 78:65–78, 1986

Olds DL, Henderson CR Jr, Tatelbaum R, et al: Improving the life-course development of socially disadvantaged mothers: a randomized trial of nurse home visitation. Am J Public Health 78:1436–1445, 1988

Olds D[L], Pettit LM, Robinson J, et al: Reducing risks for antisocial behavior with a program of prenatal and early childhood home visits. J Community Psychol 26:65–83, 1998

O'Leary KD: Physical aggression in intimate relationships can be treated within a marital context under certain circumstances. Journal of Interpersonal Violence 11:450–452, 1996

O'Leary KD, Cascardi M: Physical aggression in marriage: a developmental analysis, in The Developmental Course of Marital Dysfunction. Edited by Bradbury TN. New York, Cambridge University Press, 1998, pp 343–374

O'Leary KD, Jacobson NS: Partner relational problems with physical abuse, in DSM-IV Sourcebook, Vol 3. Edited by Widiger TA, Frances AJ, Pincus HA, et al. Washington, DC, American Psychiatric Association, 1997, pp 673–692

O'Leary KD, Curley A, Rosenbaum A, et al: Assertion training for abused wives: a potentially hazardous treatment. J Marital Fam Ther 11:319–322, 1985

O'Leary KD, Vivian D, Malone J: Assessment of physical aggression against women in marriage: the need for multimodal assessment. Behavioral Assessment 14:5–14, 1992

Oliveri ME, Reiss D: A theory-based empirical classification of family problem-solving behavior. Fam Process 20:409–418, 1981

Oliveri ME, Reiss D: Family concepts and their measurements: things are seldom what they seem. Fam Process 23:33–48, 1984

Pasternak RE: The symptom profile and two-year course of subsyndromal depression in spousally bereaved elders. Am J Geriatr Psychiatry 2:210–219, 1994

Patterson GR, DeBaryshe BD, Ramsey E: A Developmental Perspective on Antisocial Behavior. Am Psychol 44:329–335, 1989

Pike A, McGuire S, Hetherington EM, et al: Family environment and adolescent depression and antisocial behavior: a multivariate genetic analysis. Dev Psychol 32:590–603, 1996

Pilkonis PA, Imber SD, Lewis P, et al: Comparative outcome study of individual, group and conjoint psychotherapy. Arch Gen Psychiatry 41:431–437, 1984

Pinshof WM, Wynne LC: The efficacy of marital and family therapy: an empirical overview, conclusions and recommendations. J Marital Fam Ther 21:585–613, 1995

Reiss D (with Neiderhiser JM, Hetherington EM, Plomin R): The Relationship Code: Deciphering Genetic and Social Influences on Adolescent Development. Cambridge, MA, Harvard University Press, 2000

Reiss D, Hetherington EM, Plomin R, et al: Genetic questions for environmental studies: differential parenting and psychopathology in adolescence. Arch Gen Psychiatry 52:925–936, 1995

Reiss D, Cederblad M, Pedersen NL, et al: Genetic probes of three theories of maternal adjustment, II: genetic and environmental influences. Fam Process 40:261–272, 2001

Rice KG, Mulkeen P: Relationships with parents and peers: a longitudinal study of adolescent intimacy. Journal of Adolescent Research 10:338–357, 1995

Rusbult CE, Bissonnette VL, Arriaga XB, et al: Accommodation processes during the early years of marriage, in The Developmental Course of Marital Dysfunction. Edited by Bradbury TN. New York, Cambridge University Press, 1998, pp 74–113

Sabelli HC: Anticholinergic antidepressants decrease marital hostility. J Clin Psychiatry 51:127–128, 1990

Sameroff AJ, Emde RN (eds): Relationship Disturbances in Early Childhood. New York, Basic Books, 1989

Schachar R, Taylor E, Wieselberg M, et al: Changes in family function and relationships in children who respond to methylphenidate. J Am Acad Child Adolesc Psychiatry 26:728–732, 1987

Segraves RT: Marriage and mental health. J Sex Marital Ther 6:187–198, 1980

Shaffer D, Gould MS, Rutter M, et al: Reliability and validity of a psychosocial axis in patients with child psychiatric disorder. J Am Acad Child Adolesc Psychiatry 30:109–115, 1991

Silk KR, Lee S, Hill EM, et al: Borderline personality disorder symptoms and severity of sexual abuse. Am J Psychiatry 152:1059–1064, 1995

Snyder D, Smith GT: Classification of marital relationships. Journal of Marriage and the Family 48:137–146, 1986

Sroufe LA: Relationships, self and individual adaptation, in Relationship Disturbances in Early Childhood. Edited by Sameroff AJ, Emde RN. New York, Basic Books, 1989, pp 70–94

Stern D: The representation of relational patterns: developmental considerations, in Relationship Disturbances in Early Childhood. Edited by Sameroff AJ, Emde RN. New York, Basic Books, 1989, pp 52–69

Straus MA: Measuring intrafamily violence and conflict: the Conflict Tactics (CT) Scale. Journal of Marriage and the Family 41:75–85, 1979

Szapocznik J, Hervis O, Rio AT, et al: Assessing change in family functioning as a result of treatment: the Structural Family Systems Rating Scale (SFSR). J Marital Fam Ther 17:295–310, 1991

Tienari P, Sorri A, Lahti I: Interaction of genetic and psychosocial factors in schizophrenia. Acta Psychiatr Scand 71:19–30, 1985

Tienari P, Wynne LC, Moring J, et al: The Finnish adoptive family study of schizophrenia: implications for family research. Br J Psychiatry Suppl 164:20–26, 1994

Widiger TA, Frances AJ, Pincus HA, et al. (eds): DSM-IV Sourcebook, Vol 3. Washington, DC, American Psychiatric Association, 1997, pp 521–857

Williams JBW: Introduction to Section IV, The DSM-IV Multiaxial System, in DSM-IV Sourcebook, Vol 3. Edited by Widiger TA, Frances AJ, Pincus HA, et al. Washington, DC, American Psychiatric Association, 1997, pp 393–400

Wilson M, Daly M: Spousal homicide risk and estrangement. Violence Vict 8:3–16, 1993

Wolin S, Wolin SJ: The challenge model: working with strengths in children of substance-abusing parents. Child Adolesc Psychiatr Clin N Am 5:243–256, 1996

Zanarini MC, Williams AA, Lewis RE, et al: Reported pathological childhood experiences associated with the development of borderline personality disorder. Am J Psychiatry 154:1101–1106, 1997

Zero to Three: Diagnostic Classification, 0–3: Diagnostic Classification of Mental Health and Developmental Disorders of Infancy and Early Childhood. Arlington, VA, Zero to Three/National Center for Clinical Infant Programs, 1994

Index

*Page numbers printed in **boldface** type refer to tables or figures.*